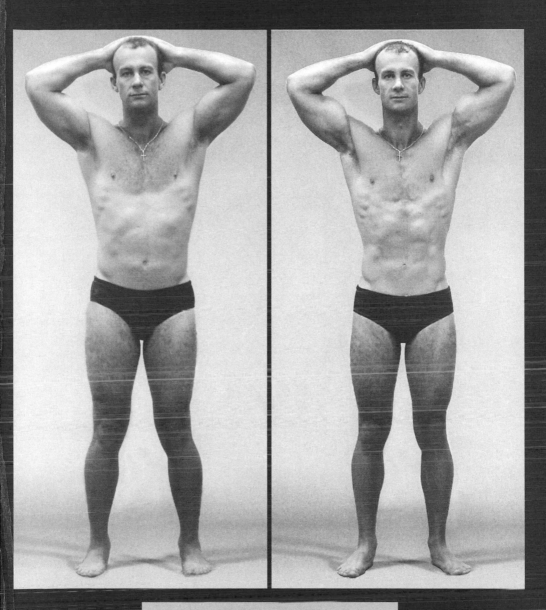

164 pounds   151 pounds

DARIN TRUTTMANN, age 29, height 5'7"
AFTER 3 WEEKS
15.5 pounds of fat loss
2.625 inches off waist
2.5 pounds of muscle gain

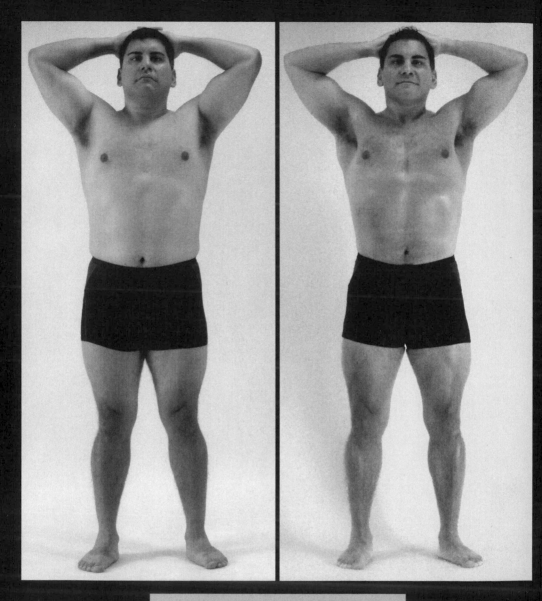

222.5 pounds   **185.5** pounds

AUSTIN DEELY, age 37, height 5'8"
AFTER 12 WEEKS
43.5 pounds of fat loss
7 inches off waist
6.5 pounds of muscle gain

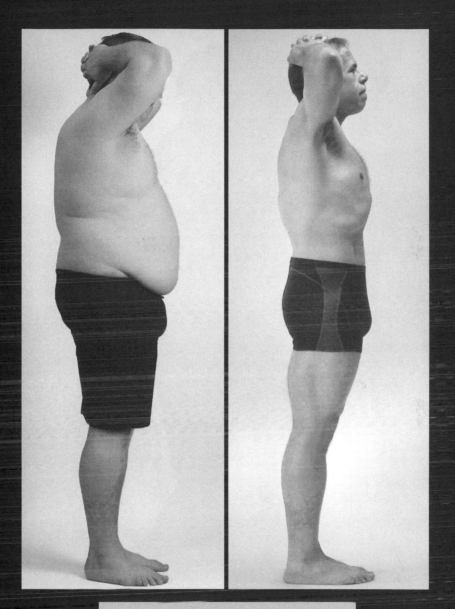

281.5 pounds   181 pounds

ANGEL RODRIGUEZ, age 48, height 5'8"
AFTER 30 WEEKS
121 pounds of fat loss
20.125 inches off waist
20.5 pounds of muscle gain

Men's Health

KILLING FAT

Use the Science of Thermodynamics to Blast Belly Bloat, Destroy Flab, and Stoke Your Metabolism

ELLINGTON DARDEN, PhD

RODALE

NEW YORK

Text copyright © 2019 by Hearst Magazines, Inc.
Before and after photographs copyright © 2019 by Ellington Darden
Exercise photographs copyright © 2019 by Hearst Magazines, Inc.

All rights reserved.
Published in the United States by Rodale Books, an imprint of the Crown Publishing Group, a division of Penguin Random House LLC, New York.
crownpublishing.com
rodalebooks.com

RODALE and the Plant colophon are registered trademarks of Penguin Random House LLC.

Men's Health is a registered trademark of Hearst Magazines, Inc.

Library of Congress Cataloging-in-Publication Data is available.

ISBN 978-1-63565-325-0
Ebook ISBN 978-1-63565-326-7

Printed in the United States of America

Exercise photographer: Footstone Photography
Exercise model: Michael Ajazi
Jacket design: Jordan Wannemacher

10 9 8 7 6 5 4 3 2 1

First Edition

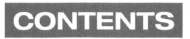
CONTENTS

Introduction: Strong, Straight Talk   **1**

PART I Killing Fat with Sizzle   9

1   The Muddle Clears Here   **11**

2   Real-World Thermodynamics   **23**

3   Backloading: Build Muscle *Fast* with 30 10–30   **31**

4   The Truth About Body Fat and Belly Bloat   **41**

5   The Killing Fat Formula for Success   **51**

PART II Eating and Exercising for Killing Fat   57

6   Food and Nutrition   **59**

7   The Eating Plan   **66**

8   The Best Type of Exercise for Fat Loss   **75**

9   The 30-10-30 Exercises   **82**

PART III Killing Fat Six-Week Programs   131

10   Before You Begin   **133**

11   The No-Fuss Eating Option   **142**

12   The Cook-at-Home Eating Option   **153**

13   Super Smoothies   **181**

14   Meal Plans   **189**

15   Positive Results from Negative Routines   **194**

16   More Fat Loss   **206**

PART IV   Specific Thermodynamic Tactics   **215**

17   Ice-Cold Drinking Water   **217**

18   Brown Fat Metabolism   **224**

19   The Cold Plunge   **230**

20   Sleep Blitzing and Bombing   **238**

PART V   Your *Killing Fat* Body for Life   **247**

21   "Tell Me Why?"   **249**

22   Patience and Overlearning   **264**

23   Jeff Shaw's Report   **275**

24   My Champions   **287**

25   Killing Fat and the Mix   **292**

BIBLIOGRAPHY   **296**

ACKNOWLEDGMENTS   **299**

INDEX   **301**

STRONG, STRAIGHT TALK

NOW IS THE PERFECT TIME TO DO SOMETHING ABOUT YOUR EXCESS FAT

THROUGHOUT LIFE, you'll find that you learn the most from the individuals who challenge you. In college, I connected with a number of innovative educators. Most of them were professors, men and women who knew their subject areas well and made learning exciting and thought-provoking.

In 1970, I encountered the smartest person I've ever met: forty-three-year-old Arthur Jones, the eventual founder of Nautilus Sports/Medical Industries and pioneer in the field of physical exercise. Jones was not a college professor. In fact, he had barely finished the ninth grade. "I always felt that quitting school in the ninth grade was one of the biggest mistakes I've ever made in my life," Jones boldly told a seminar group in Florida. "I should have quit in the sixth grade."

Jones had a wry wit, and he often made comments that were both meaningful and funny.

His wisdom was a result of rare genetics and a curiosity about the world. Nine members of his family were medical doctors. Before the age of ten, he had read hundreds of medical books. Studying on his own, he became fluent in eight languages. By the time he turned fifteen, he had visited every state in the union and parts of Canada, Mexico, and British Honduras—and he had been in and out of trouble in most of them.

Jones mentioned that during his teenage years and early twenties, at a height of 5 feet 7 inches and a weight of 160 pounds, he had been in more than seventy-five fistfights—and never lost a single one. "But often, to save my own ass"—he smiled—"I had to get out of town *fast.*"

When I first met Jones, he showed me a large, steel, rectangular, multifaceted exercise device, which led to the development of Nautilus strength-training machines. Jones was hesitant to get involved in the exercise business because of its notorious array of shady characters, half-baked advertisements, and worthless contraptions.

Jones's machines, however, were uniquely worthwhile. If you were willing to put forth intense effort, they stimulated muscular size and strength . . . quickly. They worked by providing full-range exercise, as opposed to the partial-range movement supplied by free weights.

Expand and Share

I worked with Jones for thirty-seven years, and together we researched and wrote more than two million words recognizing the true science of exercise, nutrition, muscle, and fat. I learned much from his guidance, his experience, and the research he supported through Nautilus Sports/Medical Industries.

Jones died in 2007, at age eighty. Several months before he died, he told me to *stop* depending on him. "Move forward," he declared. "You are now the mentor—the mentor you, in fact, required at an earlier age.

"Once around is enough. You no longer need my help. Let me die. Stop thinking about me."

"Arthur," I countered, "I cannot forget you and what I've learned."

"Remember the exercise basics and remember the meaningful times," he said in a fatigued voice. "But don't dwell there. Make mistakes, unlearn, relearn, and expand. Then share your findings and stories.

"Now get out, leave me alone, go home."

That was the Arthur Jones I knew, admired, and followed. He could be blunt, rough, and rude. But he was a master teacher . . . and he was still teaching me. He was right. It was time to move on, to move forward.

Some eleven years later, here I am composing at my computer. I've made plenty of mistakes, and I've expanded and relearned. I've tested and retested dozens of new guidelines and new techniques related to exercising and eating. I've made a lot of progress—even some breakthroughs. It's time to share.

Very few popular books are published for men who want to get rid of fat. The vast majority of the weight loss market is geared to women. *Killing Fat*, however, is specifically designed for the readers of *Men's Health*. It integrates scientific facts, truths, and challenges—nothing is sugarcoated.

Getting rid of significant adipose tissue is difficult, and keeping it off for longer than three years is even more difficult. At the end of the three-year mark, 99 percent of men who have lost significant weight have regained their lost fat.

Such difficulties can be studied and conquered. That's exactly what Jones and I were able to achieve from decades of discoveries with athletes and non-athletes, and what I will now share with you.

I've got a feeling that the roll of fat around your waist has been gradually telling you, *Do something. Get motivated. Shrink me, please.*

I can tell there has never been a better time to move into action against your excess fat.

I have sound answers and serious solutions. Plus, a program that will target successfully your problem areas.

Research and Results

This is "not my first rodeo," as the old saying goes. It's not my first book, either. For more than three decades, I've teamed with Joe Cirulli, who owns and operates Gainesville Health & Fitness, the largest health club in the world, in Gainesville, Florida.

Cirulli was an early Arthur Jones fan and a big believer in strength training. By 1980, Cirulli's club had one hundred Nautilus machines in constant use. From 1985 until 2018, I tested, trained, and dieted 1,209 of his Gainesville members. Many of their names, measurements, photos, and results have been reported in twelve published manuals.

When I was director of research for Nautilus Sports/Medical Industries from 1973 through 1992, I personally trained 524 athletes and non-athletes on six-week programs. More recently, from 2000 through 2018, I supervised another seventy-nine people through intensive coaching in my home gym in Windermere, Florida.

Thus, over forty-five years, I have collected the before-and-after pictures, evaluations, and workout records of and interviews with 1,812 individuals. This archive of data and experience underlies each chapter of this how-to program.

In part III of *Killing Fat*, I'll share my updated six-week eating and exercise plan. Bar none, the Killing Fat programs are the best courses of action for body leanness that I've ever designed, tested, and offered.

Killing is a strong word, especially in the title of this book. In this context, it means causing the death of excessive fat or adipose tissue. Other than surgery, which I don't often recommend, you can't really "kill" your fat cells. As you'll learn in chapter 1, you can only *transfer* them out of your body.

But if you apply the guidelines in this book, you can keep your transferred fat from ever returning to your system. Thus, in a broader sense, you will in fact be *killing* your unwanted fat with certain thermodynamic tactics.

For this book, *thermodynamics* is defined as how heat and cold affect human physiology, especially as it connects to fat cell shrinkage and transfer. Thermodynamics will soon become your new best friend. Plus, a recently uncovered concept called thermodynamic synergy will be revealed in chapter 1. Look for it.

In chapters 8 and 9, you'll understand and learn how to apply a new, muscle-building technique called 30–10–30. This new technique involves accentuation of the negative, or lowering, phase of a strength-training repetition. Mastering such style makes a faster, deeper, and more thorough inroad into your starting level of strength.

The end result is the stimulation of growth hormone, which causes your muscles to overcompensate, require more sleep, and get bigger and stronger. You'll see and feel more and more muscle being added to your body on a week-by-week basis.

But that's not all. Your expanding contractile tissue will radiate extra heat and help you melt and transfer more fat. Growing muscles are an important aspect in the process of killing fat.

If you are a woman, please don't be afraid of getting muscles that are too big. Recently, I supervised thirty-four women through my six-week program. The average muscle gain per woman was 5 pounds—that's 5 pounds in six weeks. Each of the thirty-four women appreciated their muscles and wanted more.

A similar group of twenty-one men, under the same conditions, added an average of 8.83 pounds of muscle to each of their physiques. That's almost 9 pounds of solid muscle, which is 1.48 pounds per week for six consecutive weeks. Such gains can change the way you look, feel, and act.

Negative-accentuated training and 30–10–30 are potent sources of muscle-building stimulation—and you'll get all the details in this course.

Shooting from the Hip

Whether you want a significantly smaller midsection, or just more muscle and less fat, it will all be carefully described in this book.

WARNING: Getting rid of pounds and inches from your waist and throughout your body requires *discipline*. Ditto for the efficient stimulation of muscular growth. These processes demand *hard work*.

Have you ever accomplished anything meaningful in your life that didn't demand focus and discipline? Probably not.

I find that people accept hard work—if *they see results in a short time*. You've already seen the before-and-after photos up front. You'll want to thumb through the rest of the book and view the others. There are thirty-eight sets in total. All these people accepted the reality of hard work and paid the price. Be sure to study the comparison pictures.

Challenge Yourself with High, but Realistic, Expectations

With Killing Fat, some individuals can shed 15 pounds of fat and lose 3.5 inches off their waists in the first two weeks. Think about this: *In the next two weeks, wouldn't you like to drop 15 pounds?*

Continuing the program for six weeks, a focused man can expect to lose 29 pounds of fat and 6 inches off his belly. A motivated woman (chapters 11, 12, and 14 adapt the program for females) can expect to remove 17 pounds of fat and 4½ inches off her middle. Those numbers, in fact, are from recent Killing Fat group averages of twenty-one men and thirty-four women.

After six weeks, if you still have excess fat to remove, you simply repeat the program in a similar manner. You'll get all the details in chapter 16.

Please look at the front cover. There's a red circle in the upper right corner, surrounding a sentence that reads: *Lose Up to 40 Pounds in Just 6 Weeks!* Most publishers of weight loss books select the dieter who did the best in a series of trials, and hype that unnamed person's results on the cover with a similar headline . . . *Lose up to X pounds quickly!*

"Up to" always precedes the number, even though that number is typically two or three times that of the losses of the other dieters. There is no mention of averages, because they are much less than anticipated and few readers would be influenced by such small numbers.

I take my numbers seriously in the Killing Fat program. After six weeks, I had four individuals who lost 50 pounds or more, eight men who dropped at least 40 pounds, and twenty-three people who lost 30 pounds or more. You'll see the actual names, numbers, and before-and-after photos of these folks throughout the book.

On the front cover, I feel justified in affirming a high, but realistic, expectation since eight men have achieved that goal:

Lose up to
40 pounds of fat
in just 6 weeks

GET READY TO:
- Cut maximum pounds and inches, fast.
- Pump up your attention-getting muscles.
- Add thermodynamics to your lifestyle.
- Forge visual impact throughout your body.
- Transfer and finally destroy your excessive fat.

Gentlemen and ladies, start your engines . . . It's fat-killing time!

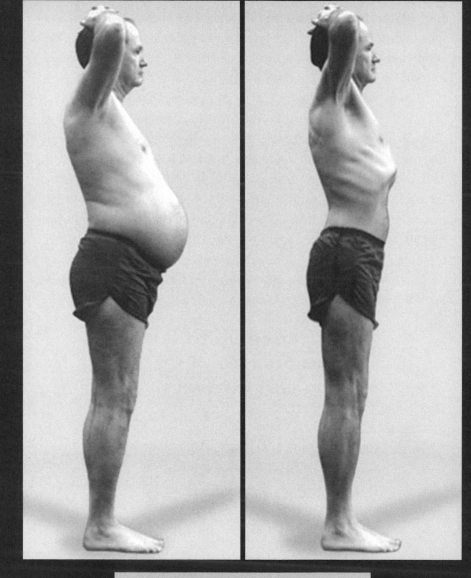

182.5 pounds   **144.5** pounds

KEN HOWELL, age 59, height 5'6"
AFTER 14 WEEKS
45.75 pounds of fat loss
10.75 inches off waist
7.75 pounds of muscle gain

Part I

KILLING FAT WITH SIZZLE

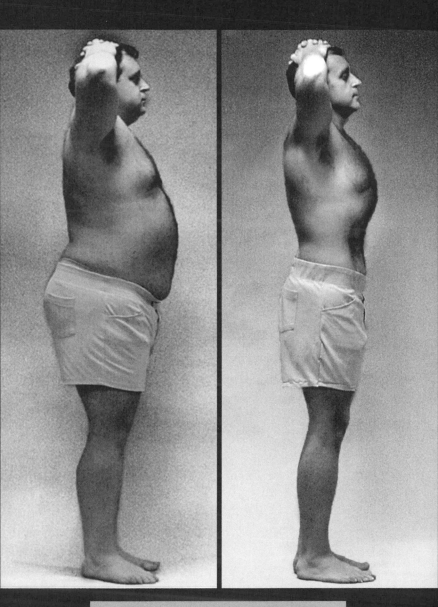

306 pounds   **195** pounds

LARRY FREEDMAN, age 29, height 5'11"
AFTER 18 WEEKS
116.5 pounds of fat loss
15.5 inches off waist, **11.125** inches off hips
5.5 pounds of muscle gain

1

THE MUDDLE CLEARS HERE

THERMODYNAMICS, SCIENCE, AND A SECRET

YOU **WANT TO** lose fat. You want to get it off *fast*. And you want it to stay off permanently, right?

I hear you. Over the last fifty years, I've tested, modified, retested, added and subtracted, and finally developed a program that's designed to deliver those results.

With a practical understanding of thermodynamics, you'll learn how to bomb, blast, and finally kill your excess body fat.

The program starts with a two-week segment, with women consuming 1,400 calories a day and men consuming 1,600 calories a day. Fourteen days can make a huge difference in the way your body feels and looks. You need focus and compliance to do what the following folks did in only two weeks.

14 POUNDS OR MORE OF FAT LOSS IN 14 DAYS

Bob Smith: 19 pounds

Larry Freedman: 17.75 pounds

Angel Rodriguez: 16.5 pounds

Javier Woody: 15.25 pounds

Storm Roberts: 15 pounds

Allison Spratt: 14.25 pounds

Travis Hastay: 14 pounds

You're going to meet all these folks and become familiar with their success stories in *Killing Fat*.

My objective for you is to get a flying start with a significant bang, to get rid of up to a pound of unneeded fat a day—just as these individuals did.

To master this undertaking requires that you harness the science of thermodynamics. Helping you grasp thermodynamics merits a brief examination of some of the teachings of Albert Einstein and Carl Sagan.

Albert Einstein and Thermodynamics

Albert Einstein was the most influential physicist of the twentieth century. He was born in Germany in 1879 and died in Princeton, New Jersey, in 1955. In 1905, he earned a PhD from the University of Zurich, and in that same year he published four groundbreaking research papers, which brought him great notoriety in the academic world.

Einstein became a professor at the University of Bern and then moved to the University of Prague for two years, and finally back to the University of Zurich, where he became a full professor. The subjects he taught were analytical mechanics and thermodynamics. For a number of years, Einstein directed much of his attention to thermodynamics and helped refine the first law of thermodynamics. All this helped him win the 1921 Nobel Prize in Physics.

The first law of thermodynamics states that energy can be *transformed*, but cannot be *created* or *destroyed*. Energy is safeguarded, maintained, and conserved over time. Einstein's famous $E = mc^2$ is still uncontestable in the confirmation of the law of conservation of energy.

In scientific research, there are guesses, theories, and hypotheses that must be tested, analyzed, rejected, retested, reanalyzed, accepted, and then repeated before that hypothesis is said to be proved. Then, after many years—and much replication—that long-standing proof may be recognized as a law. A law, therefore, represents *an unwavering relationship of events under a specific set of conditions*.

Over one hundred years ago, Einstein and other scientists authenticated and verified the law of conservation of energy. In other words, energy, fat, heat, and calories are conserved over time. And now we're using this principle to transfer body fat.

Transferring Body Fat by Albert Einstein

Fat-loss knowledge and practices must be established by examining the physics of heat and the transfer of it. Transfers, according to any thermodynamic primer, begin with the sun.

Animals and humans have no way to capture the sun's energy directly. But plants can trap solar energy by using it to combine carbon dioxide and water. The product of this combination is a hydrated carbon (carbohydrate). This basic science is as follows:

Plants grow by sun + air + soil + water.

Animals grow by consuming plants.

Humans grow by eating plants (carbohydrates) and
animals (proteins and fats).

Carbohydrates, proteins, and fats supply units of
heat energy called **calories**.

Calories are stored in the body primarily in **fat** cells.

Humans use fat calories and transfer heat from them
through their skin, urine, and exhaled carbon dioxide to
plants, **animals**, and the **environment**.

Once you understand the above relationship, the following circular applications are appropriate:

Heat = Calories = Fat = Energy = Heat

For fat loss: Heat out must be **more** than heat in.

For fat stabilization: Heat out must be **equal** to heat in.

For fat gain: Heat out must be **less** than heat in.

Thank You, Dr. Einstein and Other Scientists

The clarity of Einstein's equations is powerful. Thermodynamics works. It applies in California, New York, Florida, and Nebraska. It succeeds in Mexico, Europe, Africa, and China. It functions on the moon, Mars, and Planet X. But within that simplicity, there are aspects that must be considered and applied.

Back in 1854, Lord Kelvin—and later other scientists, including William Rankine, Max Planck, Einstein, and E. A. Guggenheim—proved that energy cannot be created or destroyed, only transferred. Once again, this is known as the first law of thermodynamics. In other words, you can't really lose any of those four interchangeable concepts—heat, calories, fat, and energy—you can only transfer them.

As such, you'll notice that throughout this book I use *transfer* and *lose* to mean the same thing.

For transfer to make complete sense, the word *calorie* needs defining.

Calorie Defined

Energy from food as well as activity is typically measured as heat and expressed as calories. A calorie (*kilocalorie* is actually the more appropriate term) is the amount of heat it takes to raise the temperature of 1 liter of water by 1 degree centigrade. To help you visualize this, 100 calories would raise the temperature of 1 liter (approximately 1 quart) of water from freezing to boiling. A calorie, therefore, is a unit of temperature measure. It is used to express the energy value of food or the energy required by the body to perform a given task.

The calories contained in the vast majority of the food supply sold within the United States have been determined by scientific studies and are based on:

1 gram of carbohydrate = 4 calories

1 gram of fat = 9 calories

1 gram of protein = 4 calories

Millions of foods have been calculated and labeled. For example:

1 extra-large egg = 92 calories

1 medium banana = 93 calories

4 Chick-fil-A Chick-n-Strips = 470 calories

Wendy's Chocolate Frosty = 340 calories

Common physical activities have also been tested in heat-sensing chambers. For example, a 180-pound man would burn the following calories in one hour of:

Cycling (10 mph) = 327 calories

Weight training = 490 calories

Basketball, shooting baskets = 368 calories

Playing tennis = 572 calories

One ounce of fat on your body contains 219 calories. Sixteen ounces, or 1 pound, supplies 3,500 calories of heat energy.

The circular science of *heat = calories = fat = energy = heat* applies equally to intake and output.

The standard thermodynamic principle of getting rid of fat is to cut calories, produce energy, burn fat, and transfer heat to the environment. Then repeat and transfer again and again.

Killing Fat Adds to the Transfer

You might be wondering exactly where the fat goes when it leaves your body. As we've discussed, when you lose fat, you transfer the energy stored in fat cells out of your body and into the environment.

A slightly different response can be found in the December 16, 2014, issue of the *British Medical Journal*. In a study of how energy is metabolized, researchers Ruben Meerman and Andrew Brown traced the pathways of atoms of energy exiting the body. The complete oxidation of a single triglyceride molecule involves many enzymes and biochemical steps, but after lengthy calculations, Meerman and Brown concluded that triglycerides stored in fat cells are primarily excreted by the lungs through respiration. Stored fat is unlocked through chemical reactions to power your body, including during exercise, and it exits the body in your exhaled breath.

According to Meerman and Brown, when a person loses 20 pounds of fat (triglycerides), 16.8 pounds are exhaled as warm carbon dioxide (CO_2), and the remaining 3.2 pounds are excreted as warm water (H_2O), primarily in the urine and sweat. But, the researchers cautioned, body fat does not shrink quickly.

Applying the standard reduced-calorie-eating/increased-calorie-burn exercising formula, they recommend 1 pound of fat loss per week. Thus, it would take twenty weeks for the average person to lose 20 pounds of fat.

On the other hand, my Killing Fat formula speeds up the fat-loss process to the degree that many of my test panelists lose an average of 4 pounds of fat each week, which equates to 32 pounds of fat loss in eight weeks. That's four times the fat loss in 40 percent of the time suggested by Meerman and Brown.

To improve the calories-in and calories-out processes, the Killing Fat program incorporates the following practices:

- A simple carbohydrate-rich eating plan that gradually decreases calories after each two-week segment. A key guideline is to eat six small meals per day.
- Two 30-minute strength-training workouts per week that involve a new negative-accentuated technique called 30–10–30. Each recommended exercise is performed with a slow 30-second lowering, followed by 10 faster-speed repetitions, followed by a final 30-second lowering. This negative-accentuated style makes a deeper inroad into your body's starting strength, which in turn triggers the release of at least six hormones that help with fat loss and muscle gain.
- Superhydration (sipping 1 gallon of ice-cold water continuously throughout the day) to accelerate calorie burn and assist fat loss.
- Heat and cold transfer, brown fat reconditioning, the cold plunge, and extra rest and sleep.

If you want to get started immediately on the initial two-week segment, you can turn to chapter 10 and review the important steps you should take before you begin. But I'd rather see you take a little time and familiarize yourself with the science behind the Killing Fat program in parts II and IV.

Carl Sagan and Science

Carl Sagan was born in 1934 and died in 1996. Early on, Sagan developed a keen sense of both wonder and skepticism—which are necessary for the cohabiting modes of thought that are central to the scientific method.

Sagan was valedictorian of his New Jersey high school at age sixteen. He continued his education at the University of Chicago, where he earned four degrees, including a PhD in astronomy and astrophysics.

In 1980 Sagan cowrote and narrated *Cosmos: A Personal Voyage*, a thirteen-part PBS television series. This show became the most widely watched series in the history of public television and was seen by at least five hundred million people across sixty different countries. His bestselling book *Cosmos* was published to accompany the series.

Sagan frequently wrote about people's vulnerability toward quackery and hoodwink—not only in the subject of outer space and all its buzz—but also in the marketing of fat-loss information. He feared that in the future, more and more people were going to slide, almost without noticing, back into ancient times of mental and physical ignorance and superstition.

"Modern science must supply answers," Sagan believed. "If we've been bamboozled long enough"—which directly applies to the bestselling low-carbohydrate eating plans dating back to the publication of *Calories Don't Count* in 1961 and continuing into 2018 with diets like South Beach, Atkins, paleo, and ketogenic—"we tend to reject any evidence of the bamboozle." In other words, the same-old misleading, not-scientific information, if it is repeated for forty years by different authors under new titles, becomes the *new truth*.

As a nation, 75 percent of us are overweight, a figure that's been stable for the last ten years. It's obvious that the millions of antiscientific weight loss books sold each year are not a positive contribution to our nation's leanness. We must learn, in our book selections, how to separate *deep truths* from *deep nonsense.*

Sagan noted that the simplest definition of science is "the search for rules." He believed that people who looked at everyday experiences as a muddled jumble of events with no predictability and no regularity were in grave danger. The vast universe that Sagan described in his books and videos belonged to people whose lives were governed by principles, rules, and guidelines.

Sagan understood the first law of thermodynamics . . . and so do I.

Clearing the Muddle

While I don't have all the laws about fat loss figured out, I have plenty of experience in supervising groups of overfat men and women as they strive to achieve leaner, stronger bodies. In the process of doing that for fifty years, I've assembled meaningful guidelines related to losing fat, building muscular size and strength, and the maintenance of both.

Thermodynamics remains the inadequately told and poorly accepted principle for losing fat. The scientifically proven key to lasting success is to fire up the body and not shut it down. It's important to understand that there's a difference between *weight* loss and *fat* loss. Thermodynamics is concerned with fat and transfer.

Remember, fat loss has to involve thermodynamics, and *all calories count.* When you eliminate carbohydrates in your diet, the fats and proteins you eat in their place do not have special qualities that cause faster fat loss. There is no hard-core scientific evidence to support the notion that the source of the calorie—not the calorie itself—is the key factor in becoming leaner. Low-carbohydrate dieting is not based on any law.

On the other hand, low-*calorie* dieting is based primarily on the first law of thermodynamics.

"I Feel Like a Man with a Brand-New Body"

One person who took thermodynamics, fat, and transfer personally was Larry Freedman. Freedman was a member of the Sheriff's Office of Alachua County, Florida, when I met him. Freedman was the heaviest trainee in his group of ten adults. He weighed 306 pounds and was 5 feet 11 inches tall, with a waist measurement of 52.625 inches. In spite of his mass, Freedman was the most motivated in his group.

At that time, Freedman dramatically shattered the individual record for fat loss. During the first six weeks, he lost 52.75 pounds of fat. Eighteen weeks (or three back-to-back six-week programs) later, Freedman was down 116.5 pounds. See Larry's photos on page 10.

He also lost 15.5 inches off his waist, 11.125 inches off his hips, and 15.375 inches off his thighs. Such decreases made huge positive differences in his mental and physical health, as well as his social life.

"The thermodynamics and the science behind the program," Freedman said, "are what sealed the deal for me. I knew science would not let me down, and it didn't.

"I feel like a man with a brand-new body."

Wouldn't you like to be included in Larry Freedman's exclusive group of ecstatic people who've lost at least 14 pounds in fourteen days?

Isn't it time you embraced thermodynamics and science? They can be your tickets to a brand-new body.

The Secret Revealed

April 4, 2018: "Dr. Darden, compared to the other published studies on fat loss, why do your subjects get significantly better results?" asked James Fisher, PhD, a British exercise physiologist from Southampton

Solent University. This well-read man had just examined Larry Freedman's before-and-after pictures and measurements, as well as others from my listing on page 12.

Then he asked: "What's your secret?"

I paused briefly and replied, "There's no secret. It's all based on science and the correct application of it."

This young physiologist was frustrated and seemed to feel somewhat snubbed by my answer. "There must be an unrecognized factor in your rescarch," Fisher said, shaking his head.

MAY 1, 2018: As I rework a section in this book, I begin reflecting on thermodynamics, Fisher's comment about an unrecognized factor, and how to edit chapter 25.

The success of my Killing Fat program involves the transformation of heat, but it's more, much more than basic thermodynamics. Suddenly, there's a flash of swirling light inside my head and I see two words:

Thermodynamic Synergy

I'm now keenly focused as I read through my manuscript of chapter 25.

On the second page, I examine a graphic I call Circles of Synergy. I visualize that these four interconnecting circles—which enclose a smaller Killing Fat circle and are surrounded by a much bigger circle—are misnamed. My circles should be called . . . thermodynamic synergy.

Thermodynamic synergy most definitely includes numerous collaborations and interactions.

This new unification, I think, is more complete, and I'm seeing it differently for the first time. Yet, for at least six years, all the information has been there in plain sight. I just failed to connect the dots.

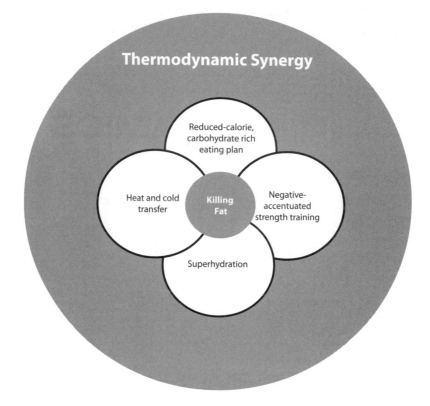

I hesitate to call the idea a secret. But, in fact, it is just that.

I have written about synergy, about $1 + 1 + 1 + 1 = 16$ (see chapter 5). The Centers for Disease Control (CDC) recommend a healthy fat loss of 1 to 2 pounds per week. Compared to the CDC's maximum of 2 pounds per week, many of my trainees are achieving 3.5 times those results. In fact, my new illustration, above, reveals that with the expanded synergy added to the mix, a few of my test panelists are raising the bar to four times the CDC's recommendations. The *why* is the secret, a secret that needs sharing.

So prepare yourself. Throughout *Killing Fat*, you're going to hear more about thermodynamic synergy.

2

REAL-WORLD THERMODYNAMICS

SOLUTIONS AND FIRE

Why Americans Are Fat

Here are the issues many Americans face:

- We've been blitzed by a complex array of eating advice focusing on fat grams, antioxidants, gluten sensitivity, veganism, grass fed, lectins, sugar-free, junk meals, supplements, and health foods. Such advice hasn't worked for the majority of fat people. Although we are consuming more low-fat and sugar-free foods than we did twenty years ago, we have compensated by eating more of everything else as well. As a result, most adults add 1 pound of fat to their bodies per year and accumulate a large amount of flab around their midsections.
- The leisure activities of most people increasingly revolve around computers, social media, movies, and other passive entertainment. As a consequence, most adults lose .5 pound of muscle per year, which causes a yearly 0.5 percent decline in metabolic rate.
- Even with all the media emphasis on the physical fitness boom of the last three decades, the end result has been a bust. Millions

of people have been injured from exercise and sports, and even more have received *no results*. Statistics show that fewer than 10 percent of adults do anything classified as *vigorous* exercise even two or three times per week.

- Research indicates that as most people age, they become dehydrated. This dryness occurs throughout the body: skin, hair, internal organs, bones, muscles, and even fatty tissues. Such dehydration can progress unnoticed for years. Even mild dehydration emphasizes the gradual loss of muscle and the gradual gain of fat.
- With the rise of the internet, more bad information exists today than ever before concerning eating and exercising.

Finding Solutions

So how do we solve these issues?

Complex dietary guidelines that lead to overconsumption of calories and the increase of body fat: People need specific guidelines that tell them exactly what to eat at each meal. Six small meals a day teach portion control, facilitate appetite regulation, and accelerate the dropping of pounds and inches.

Loss of muscle mass: Negative-accentuated strength training—highlighted by the new 30–10–30 technique—efficiently builds muscles, whether they are atrophied, plateaued, or unused. Negative-accentuated training involves the use of dumbbells, barbells, home equipment, and heavy-duty health-club machines.

Unsafe and unproductive exercise: Many types of exercise can become unsafe and unproductive when performed in a fast, jerky manner. The safest and most productive form of strength training involves doing the negative phase of each repetition slowly and smoothly.

Dehydration: The cure for dehydration involves more than gulping down extra water. It entails the systematic and progressive sipping of 1 gallon of ice-cold water each day. "Superhydration" is the name I've given this process.

Too much misleading information: A carefully organized, six-week program with daily guidelines combats misinformation and yields fast fat transfer.

Add Fire to Your Body

Most diets are about shutting down your body, kind of like a "going out of business" sale. Cutting out major food groups, such as carbohydrates, usually leads to the loss of critical, metabolically active, lean tissue—your *muscle*. You don't need to get rid of muscle. Muscle stokes your metabolism.

The key to permanent weight reduction is to understand, initially, that F-A-T is the enemy. Your desired goal is *not* a specific number of pounds on the scale.

The answer to lasting anti-flab success is to add fire to your metabolism. I want you to fire up to lose fat—not wither down your internal systems for that self-defeating, temporary weight loss.

What does it mean to *fire up*? Firing up is forcing your body—your brain, hormones, contractile tissues, and even your adipose cells—to work for you, not against you. Stoking your metabolism is the sure way to get rid of that unwanted fat.

Again, the number of pounds your body *weighs* is not your enemy—excess fat is. It's the unhealthy and undesirable flab that you

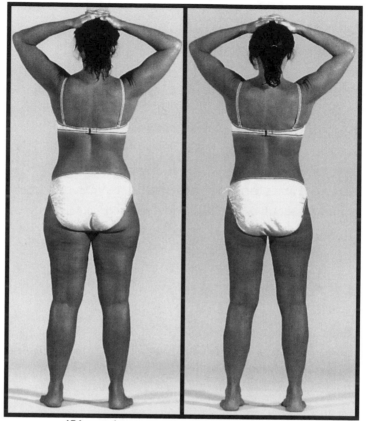

154 pounds   **134** pounds

BARRIE GAFFNEY, age 41, height 5'5"
AFTER 6 WEEKS
23.5 pounds of fat loss
5.125 inches off hips
7.875 inches off thighs
3.5 pounds of muscle gain

want to remove, and it's only by fueling and sustaining the internal heat that you can achieve long-lasting results.

Of course, you have to know how to measure and calculate the fat on your body. I have a simple measurement tool that I'll share and demonstrate in chapter 10. Using my recommended technique is a way to guarantee that your lost weight is 100 percent fat.

Muscles, Thermodynamics, and Fire

A seldom-understood part of the entire process is to *appreciate* and *cherish* your muscles. Rebuild what has atrophied and then push your contractile tissues to stronger levels. As a result, there will be intense fire in your muscles, and your physique will soon grasp the power and energy of the ageless external and internal laws referred to as *thermodynamics*.

Thermodynamics is the science behind the fire. It will help you rejuvenate your metabolism and gain the body you've always wanted.

I progressed to the Killing Fat concept of thermodynamics and thermodynamic synergy after years of working with thousands of obese subjects in diet and exercise programs. This book is the culmination of what I have learned and witnessed in the people I have trained.

TRUE OR FALSE:
95 PERCENT OF DIETERS REGAIN LOST WEIGHT WITHIN 1 YEAR

From 1960 to 2000, I remember reading multiple articles stating that 95 percent of dieters who lost significant weight would regain what they had lost within the first year. Occasionally, the number would be upped to 97, 98, or even 99 percent over the course of two, three, or five years. Were any of these figures based on actual scientific studies?

DR. ALBERT STUNKARD'S FINDINGS

According to a 1999 article in the *New York Times* by Jane Fritsch, the "95 percent" statistic was simply passed down as part of the mythology of obesity. Fritsch traced the opinion back to a non-random sample of one hundred patients treated for obesity by Dr. Albert Stunkard in New York Hospital in 1959. Dr. Stunkard concluded, "Most obese persons will not stay in treatment, most will not lose weight, and those who do lose weight, most will regain it." Then he alluded to the 95 percent figure.

Fritsch talked with Stunkard in 1999, and he admitted that his study, reported in the *Archives of Internal Medicine* forty years earlier, was very simplistic and that the hundred patients were just given a written diet and sent home. There were no attempts at behavior modification and there was little accountability, reinforcement, or follow-up. "I've been sort of surprised," Stunkard noted, "that people keep citing it."

But they did, and continue to do so.

Dr. Kelly Brownell, former director of the Rudd Center for Food Policy and Obesity, agreed that the 95 percent figure has become the most frequently quoted statement in obesity literature. "The true failure rate could be much better, or much worse," said Brownell, who is now at Duke University. "The fact is we just don't know."

KING'S COLLEGE STUDY

In 2015 Dr. Alison Fildes and colleagues at King's College London completed a huge study that was reported in the *American Journal of Public Health*. Instead of looking at the probability of people keeping the weight off, they initially examined the question: Could they get it off in the first place? The research tracked the weight of 278,982 men and women in Great Britain between 2004 and 2014 using electronic health records. All these men and women had been evaluated to be obese.

Only 1,283 men and 2,245 women in the study reached a non-obese body weight. The probability of reaching this number in one year was 1 in 210 for men and 1 in 124 for women. These numbers represented a success rate much lower than 1 percent; or, said another way, more than 99 percent of these people failed to reach a normal body weight.

It was much, much worse for the morbidly obese: the one-year rate was 1 in 1,290 for men and 1 in 677 for women, or an average failure rate of 99.99 percent.

The study also looked at the one-year rate of obese patients attaining something more reasonable: a *5-percent* reduction in body weight. For example, for a woman who weighs 180 pounds, 5 percent is 9 pounds; for a man who weighs 240 pounds, 5 percent is 12 pounds. For both groups, the weight reduction is hardly noticeable in before-and-after photos. Unfortunately, 53 percent regained this weight within two years and 78 percent had regained it within five years.

The King's College study's overall conclusions were as follows:

> *Our findings indicate that current obesity treatment strategies are failing to achieve sustained weight loss for a majority of obese patients. For morbidly obese patients, maintaining weight loss was rare and the probability of achieving normal weight was extremely low. Research to develop new and more effective approaches to obesity management is urgently required.*

MORE TRUE THAN FALSE INVOLVED

Based on the research, I would have to say it's true that about 95 percent of dieters regain their lost weight within one year. In fact, it's my opinion that 99 percent of all people who lose significant weight gain it back within three years. I tell all my trainees that if they can keep their lost fat off for three years, the process of maintenance becomes much easier.

KILLING FAT SUCCESSES: 17 TIMES
MORE LIKELY *NOT* TO REGAIN

With my Killing Fat program, 17 percent of successful participants have managed to keep their lost fat off after three years.

That's Killing Fat at 17 percent, compared to established dieting programs at 1 percent.

In other words, compared to traditional practices and results, which don't involve low-calorie eating, strength training, and superhydration, a Killing Fat trainee is 17 times more likely to have kept his or her lost fat off after three years.

It's disappointing when any of my participants regain their lost fat. Typically this occurs because a participant has stopped their high-intensity training. When that occurs, there's atrophy of the skeletal muscles that were built during the program, and resting metabolism lowers accordingly. If such a person doesn't cut back on his dietary caloric intake, the fat comes back.

A participant who is serious about losing fat and keeping it off has to apply, adapt, and maintain the Killing Fat guidelines—and keep adhering to those guidelines—for as long as he or she wants a lean, strong body.

3

BACKLOADING

BUILD MUSCLE *FAST* WITH 30-10-30

DURING A NORMAL barbell exercise, a repetition has a *front* load: the lifting or positive phase. A typical repetition also has a *back* load: the lowering or negative phase. The negative phase and backloading are fundamentally the same thing. Bodybuilders traditionally paid attention to the front load. The back load was done quickly or haphazardly, or sometimes the weight was just dropped.

Four decades ago, I discovered that the *backloading* of a repetition was much more of a trigger for muscular growth than the *frontloading*.

You are 40 percent stronger in the lowering, compared to the lifting, and heavy overloading of the negative involves more force and recruits a greater number of the larger, fast-grow muscle fibers—including those at deeper levels.

The lowering of a repetition, therefore, should never be ignored. It should be emphasized.

Every man who has worked out with a barbell has at one time thought seriously about building bigger and stronger biceps. Here's a biceps-building technique to try today that's going to knock your socks off and make you a believer in 30-10-30. Done correctly, 30-10-30 makes a deeper inroad into your existing level of strength, which will trigger several hormones that help fat loss. Again, that's the wonder of thermodynamics interacting with both building muscle and losing fat. Go into your home gym, garage, or local fitness center and grab a barbell.

The 30–10–30 Challenge

30–10–30 stands for a slow **30**-second negative repetition, followed immediately by **10** faster positive/negative repetitions with controlled turnarounds, followed by a finishing **30**-second negative repetition. The entire set takes approximately 90 seconds.

This 30–10–30 technique for the standing biceps curl is best performed with the help of a training partner who has a watch with a second hand. But you can also train without a partner by having a clock nearby, with the second hand in plain sight. You'll have to cheat a little on your first positive repetition. For now, however, let's assume you do have a training partner. Begin with a resistance on the barbell that is 80 percent of what you'd normally do for 10 repetitions. Have your training partner assist you in getting the initial repetition into the top position.

Begin the slow lowering, as your training partner calls out the seconds: 5, 10, 15, 20, 25, 30. Try to be halfway down, where your forearms are parallel to the floor, at the 15-second mark. Breathe and continue to move slowly.

At the bottom of the 30-second negative, switch to doing 10 faster positive/negative repetitions. Take about 1 second on each positive and 2 seconds on each negative movement.

After your last positive repetition, do a finishing 30-second negative, with the same 5-second guides. Note: If you've selected the resistance correctly, that final 30-second lowering should be very difficult.

Don't be surprised if you have to sit down after this 90-second set. A minute or so later, you should feel a pronounced pump in your biceps muscles—which is good.

You've just completed your first experience with 30–10–30. In chapter 9, I'll provide you with all the details and illustrations on how to plan and perform 30–10–30 routines with the recommended exercises.

Here is an example of backloading from the first person I trained using 30–10–30. His name is Jordan Rapport, and did he ever experience *fast* muscular growth.

Fast Muscular Growth

At age seventeen, Jordan Rapport built 21.25 pounds of muscle in six weeks—and he trained only one time a week. That's an average of 3.54 pounds of muscle gained per week from each workout. Each workout lasted less than 30 minutes.

"It was the spring before my senior year in high school," remembered Rapport. "I wanted to try out for the football team, but I was skinny. None of the coaches paid attention to me. My dad introduced me to Dr. Darden, and he thought I'd make a good test subject for his new program.

"I didn't know positive exercise from negative," Rapport continued, "but I did know how to follow directions. My scrawny body immediately responded to the intense lowering—and started growing, day by day. I could feel it.

"Twenty pounds of muscle made a real difference in my confidence. Next thing I know, I'm a starter on the football team, and I had an outstanding senior year. It all originated earlier from Dr. Darden's 30–10–30 concept, which literally blasted my body parts with more muscle."

Rapport will graduate from Florida State University in 2019, with a major in military science.

Since I trained Rapport in 2013, I've worked with a dozen men, all of whom have added from 10 to 20 pounds of muscle to their bodies in six weeks. (Note that Rapport, at 9.8 percent body fat, was not trying to get leaner. Thus, he did not consume a reduced-calorie diet.)

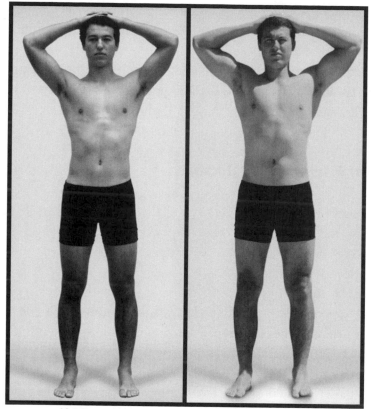

184.5 pounds   **203.3** pounds

JORDAN RAPPORT, age 17, height 6'2"
AFTER 6 WEEKS
(on muscle-building program only)
2.43 pounds of fat loss
2.5 inches added on upper arms, **3** inches on chest
4.25 inches added on thighs
21.25 pounds of muscle gain

Gradual Muscular Growth

Besides rapid enlargement, muscular growth can also be gradual and occur over six to twelve months. I've trained several teenagers who have improved in a steadier manner. Chris Medary is a young man who stands out as being the poster child for gradual growth.

In 2008, I began working with his father, Dr. Max Medary, a neuro-surgeon in Orlando, on my Intensive Coaching program. Dr. Medary lived nearby and had three boys who were several years older than my son, Tyler. Chris, Dr. Medary's oldest son, was interested in playing high school football and lacrosse and was keen to start strength training. He began training with me on a weekly basis.

At age fourteen, Chris was 5 feet 7 inches tall and weighed 143.5 pounds. Over the next year, Chris trained forty times, or approximately once every nine days. His strength increased dramatically, as did his body weight.

Within four months, Chris was doing types of workouts similar to those Jordan Rapport would eventually use. About half of Chris's exercises required a negative-accentuated style.

Chris's steady muscular growth looked like this:

June–August:	8.5 pounds
September–November:	7.125 pounds
December–February:	6.875 pounds
March–May:	8 pounds
Total gain:	**30.5 pounds** in 12 months

Over twelve months, Chris's body weight went from 143.5 pounds to 174 pounds, for a gain of 30.5 pounds. His height increased by 2 inches. Some of Chris's muscular gains were due to his normal maturation process, but we can attribute most of it to his new training program.

In 2009, as a sophomore at Lake Highland Prep in Orlando, Chris played football. During his junior and senior years, he played lacrosse exclusively, and Lake Highland Prep won the Florida state championship in 2011. Chris graduated from high school in 2012.

Today, he remains in lean condition and still weighs 174 pounds.

(Note: Chris's younger brother, Branden Medary, also went through my muscle-building program successfully in the summer of 2017, and his results are shown on page 141.)

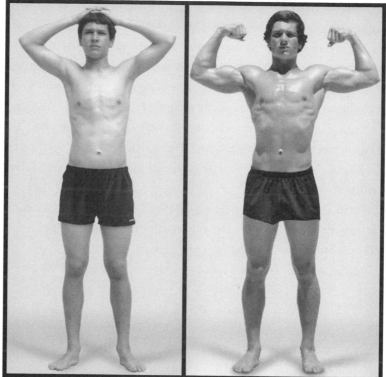

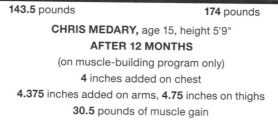

143.5 pounds   **174** pounds

CHRIS MEDARY, age 15, height 5'9"
AFTER 12 MONTHS
(on muscle-building program only)
4 inches added on chest
4.375 inches added on arms, **4.75** inches on thighs
30.5 pounds of muscle gain

How Muscle Connects to Fat Loss

If you examine samples of muscle and fat under a microscope, you'll notice that muscle has many more capillaries for blood flow than fat does. Blood flow is one reason muscle is red and fat is white. Interestingly, a pound of muscle requires approximately 37.5 calories of heat per day to live, while a pound of fat needs only 2 calories of heat. In other words, a pound of muscle burns 18.75 times as many calories as a pound of fat.

The average man has 26 pounds more muscle on his body than the average woman does. As a result, this extra muscle requires more calories each day—just to keep the muscle alive and functioning. That's one reason why men consistently lose significantly more fat per day, per week, and per month compared to women on similar diets.

The following account is about Elijah Gavarrete, age twenty, who went through my Killing Fat program in the fall of 2017. Gavarrete was 6 feet tall and very active. He was at the Gainesville Health & Fitness five days a week lifting weights and doing Spin classes. But nothing seemed to reduce his body weight. Gavarrete thought it was time for a change.

"My Body Was Confused"

"It was during Dr. Darden's introductory meeting," Gavarrete recalled, "and he discussed the difference between losing weight and losing fat. I realized that I had been confused by the terms for years. I had spent so much time working on the wrong things and not enough time focusing on my real concern: fat."

The first time I saw Gavarrete, I knew he would be great for my Killing Fat program. I could tell he cared about his health and appearance.

"I have a lot of torso fat," he noted in a serious manner to me. "I got rid of some of my belly fat over the summer, but I still have this flabby middle area—which I can't stand."

My challenge to him was as follows: "You've got to quit shutting your body down with too much lifting and Spinning. You must fire it up by stimulating your muscles to grow and allowing them time to get bigger. Eat the right foods and drink lots of water. No more five-days-a-week exercising. Instead, I want you to rest and sleep more. And use the cold plunge. These guidelines, performed seriously, will stoke your metabolism and shrink your fat cells."

I explained to Gavarrete as I measured his flexed upper arm, "You can't contract fat. That's why there's only a five-eighths-of-an-inch difference between your relaxed and contracted arm."

Then I explained to Gavarrete that he should be losing fat and only fat on a day-by-day basis. As a result, the difference between his relaxed and contracted upper-arm measurements would increase each week. On the other hand, if he were losing muscle, the difference between the two would decrease.

One goes up and the other goes down because . . . you can't contract fat. Only muscle contains contractile tissue. Fat just hangs around muscle: on top of it, behind it, and often intermingled within it.

The majority of your noncontractile fat is stored directly under your skin, with thicker layers around your midsection, hips, and thighs. When your percentage of fat is reduced, it's reduced from all over your body, not in one targeted area.

Gavarrete, with a determined look, announced, "A more muscular body is what I want to achieve—and I'll follow your details, I promise." And wow, did he ever. In six weeks, he removed 27 pounds of fat and a total of 4.5 inches from his waist, while adding 4 pounds of muscle.

"I now have a body that's leaner, stronger, and a lot more muscular, especially around the midsection," he recently told me. "I want additional muscularity . . . and I'll have it soon."

That's the way muscles are. Once you build 4 or 5 pounds of it, you always want more. And because your muscles require more calories each day, your body automatically burns more fat, and you get leaner and leaner.

Relaxed vs. Contracted Test

I designed the following test back in 1980, when I was director of research for Nautilus Sports/Medical Industries. It's more accurate to have someone do the measurements for you. Take the measurements "cold," with no warming up. Here are the techniques to apply:

- Relax the upper arm and measure the circumference midway between the elbow and the tip of the shoulder, with the arm hanging away from the body. Record the measurement to the nearest .0625 ($\frac{1}{16}$) inch.
- Contract the biceps with the upper arm parallel to the floor and measure it at right angles to the bone around the largest part of the contracted biceps. Record the measurement to the nearest .0625 ($\frac{1}{16}$) inch.
- Determine the difference between the relaxed and contracted measurements.

Gavarrete's relaxed upper arm was 14.5 inches and his contracted arm was 15.125 inches—for a difference of .625 inch. From the list below, you can see the estimated percentage of body fat was approximately 21 percent. At the end of the study, Gavarrete's measurements were 13.25 and 14.25 inches, for a difference of exactly 1 inch.

That was an improvement of .375 inch, because he had lost significant adipose tissue from all over his body, including his upper arms.

1.5-inch or more difference = 7%

1.25-inch difference = 10%

1-inch difference = 13%

.75-inch difference = 18%

.5-inch difference = 24%

Less than .5-inch difference = greater than 24%

The largest difference I've ever measured was on the arm of Casey Viator, who won AAU Mr. America in 1971. Viator's right arm was 17.125 inches relaxed and 19.3125 inches contracted—which amounted to a 2.25-inch difference.

Viator was off-the-chart lean during that time in his life.

By keeping accurate records of the difference between your relaxed and contracted arm measurements, you now have a simple way to monitor your leanness.

The Most Productive Method

As a man—young, old, or in between—you need more muscle. More muscle automatically means a smaller percentage of body fat. Extra muscle burns more calories all day and all night. Eventually that extra muscle will allow you to eat more of the foods you really like.

The best way to build extra muscle is by incorporating my new technique, 30–10–30, which is my latest—and most productive—method of backloading.

4

THE TRUTH ABOUT BODY FAT AND BELLY BLOAT

IGNORANCE IS NOT A VIRTUE

THERE IS A lot you probably don't know about body fat. In fact, some of it actually evolved to generate heat, to burn more calories under cold conditions. I'm here to tell you it's possible to activate that type of fat and ignite an extra 500 calories each day.

First, let's give that tissue we call fat a close examination. From 1970 to 2010, body fat was classified in three ways:

Subcutaneous: Fat that lies in layers directly under the skin.

Depot: Inherited fat deposited in certain areas of the body, such as the belly, hips, and upper thighs.

Essential: Fat that cushions and protects many vital organs of the body.

Approximately 50 percent of the fat stored by the average human body was subcutaneous, 40 percent was depot, and 10 percent was essential. A person could reduce subcutaneous and depot fat, but not essential fat.

In the last decade, there has been a new classification, as well as some reworked breakdowns of familiar fats. The latest science is intriguing and reveals that there are now two main categories of fat: white and brown.

White Fat: Tradition and New Classifications

White fat is composed primarily of subcutaneous and depot fats. It is our main source of long-term energy. Aside from storing calories, white fat also produces hormones like adipokinectin, which makes muscles and the liver more sensitive to the effects of insulin. It also suppresses your appetite. The trouble is, when you acquire too much white fat, your body stops making adipokinectin.

To add to the problem, fat cells also produce estrogen in both men and women, and once body-fat levels climb, so do estrogen levels. Thus, an abundance of this hormone allows the fat to get fatter.

There are several subcategories of white fat. Some are useful and some can be harmful.

Subcutaneous fat: This is the type of fat that most bodybuilders want less of to get ripped and shredded. It's also what the skinfold caliper pinches when it measures your body fat. It doesn't affect your health negatively, and it might even be advantageous, depending on where it's located. "Flab" is another name for flaccid subcutaneous fat, especially around the waist.

Thigh and butt fat: At one time, this was labeled "depot" fat. This type of fat is more likely to plague women and is the cause of the "pear" body shape. There is actually some emerging evidence that pear-shaped women are protected against metabolic diseases, at least compared to big-bellied men. Once women hit menopause, they tend to lose this protection as they shift to storing fat in their abdomen instead of on their butt and thighs.

Visceral fat: This is adipose tissue that burrows among and wraps itself around your abdominal organs. If you've got a big waist or big belly, you most certainly have some visceral fat. Lots of visceral fat drives up the risk of heart disease and stroke. Visceral fat also seems to play a bigger role than other subcategories in increasing insulin resistance, and causing diabetes as a result.

Belly fat: This type of fat is both subcutaneous and visceral. Where it shifts from being one type to another is almost impossible to tell without a CT scan, but that's a costly, impractical, and probably useless differentiation. Suffice it to say that too much belly fat—more than a 40-inch waistline for men or a 35-inch waistline for women—puts you at increased risk for heart disease, stroke, and diabetes.

Essential fat: Still a subclassification, this fat is stored in small protective amounts in your organs, bones, muscles, nerves, and even around your eyes. Women have more than men, and you never get rid of your essential fat.

Brown Fat: Something New

Only in the last ten years has brown fat emerged as a talked-about topic. Brown fat is rich with energy-producing mitochondria that are brownish in color. The mitochondria feed on droplets supplied by white fat to create energy and, as a by-product, heat.

Newborn babies, during their first year, don't have the ability to shiver in the cold. But they do have brown fat around their neck and shoulders, which allows all their mitochondria-rich cells to produce warmth.

Scientists used to think that as kids grew older, their deposits of brown fat dissipated. But in the last decade, they have discovered that adults do have deep levels of brown fat around the neck, shoulders, and spine.

Furthermore, scientists have found that it's possible to rev up the activity of brown fat, plus make some white fat act like brown fat—and in doing so, burn several hundred extra calories a day.

In one 2012 study, scientists had men sit in cold suits that circulated water cooled to a temperature of 64.4°F for three hours. The volunteers burned an extra 250 calories per man compared to what they would have burned just sitting there at normal room temperature.

You can make white fat cells turn "beige" by using a similar cold protocol, without the cold suits. For six weeks, Japanese researchers had twelve men with lower-than-average amounts of brown fat sit in rooms that had been cooled to 63°F for two hours a day. At the conclusion of the experiment, the men's bodies had "browned" some of their white fat and as a result were burning an average of 289 extra calories a day.

Naturally, the methods described above are a bit impractical. But you can certainly decide this winter to keep your thermostat as low as you can tolerate and wear clothing that is more appropriate for warm weather. Doing so will activate at least some of your brown fat.

In chapter 19, I'll present the cold-plunge protocol that many of my test panelists applied successfully at Gainesville Health & Fitness.

Fat Cells: The Good Guys

Fat is hated, yes. But you'd never want to eliminate it entirely from your body. Even the leanest people in the world have 5 percent body fat. In fact, fat is a critical organ that has more influence on your body than you might believe. For example:

- Fat cells pack together so efficiently that 20,000 calories weighs only 5 pounds.
- Fat cells are used for producing warmth, to insulate our organs, and as a messenger for our immune system.

- Brain cells are dependent on fat. Parts of your brain cells are sheathed in a substance called myelin, which is made of fat.
- Fat cells make a hormone, leptin, that allows the brain to regulate appetite.
- Fat, through leptin, enhances the size and function of the brain.
- Fat influences sexual maturation, menstruation, and pregnancy. A certain amount of fat is needed for reproduction.
- Fat and bone influence each other with hormones. Fat increases bone and bone increases fat through a reciprocal process.
- Fat can help sustain body functions during sickness and recovery.

Fat Cells: The Bad Guys

You need a small amount of fat on your body, but too much of it can cause problems.

- Fat cells have the unique ability to store fat—lots of it. They can expand their volume to more than 1,000 times normal size by pushing other cell contents off to the side.
- In the case of crowded fat cells, the cells no longer respond well to insulin, a hormone produced in the pancreas that normally helps your body turn glucose into energy. The sugars and fats circulating in your bloodstream start piling up in places they don't belong: the arteries, liver, and intestines.
- Fat throughout the gut is the most dangerous kind, and high levels of it correlate directly to diabetes, heart disease, and high cholesterol.
- As you get older, in your forties, the percentage of fat on your body increases and becomes more troublesome. Fat begins to accumulate on the belly and lower back of men and the buttocks, thighs, and breasts of women.
- In your fifties and sixties, you are typically at your heaviest and have the most difficult time keeping fat in check.

- Fat begets fat. Studies show that fat can grow right back after liposuction, and not necessarily in the same places.

Characteristics of Fat Cells

Fat cells are like balloons. They have the capacity to inflate many times over normal from excessive lipid material, or to deflate to almost empty sacks if dietary restrictions are properly applied.

The largest of the cells have the diameter of a human hair, which means the balloons are extremely small. As a result, adults have *billions* of fat cells throughout their systems. Scientists have taken fat samples from all over the body, counted, and totaled them—with the help of extrapolation. These calculations vary greatly according to individual genetics. The numbers, however, range from a low of 10 billion to a high of 250 billion. A person with a minimum number of fat cells has a lower probability of being obese, compared to a person with a high number of fat cells.

There are significant gender differences. It is estimated that the average woman in the United States has approximately 42 billion fat cells. The average man has about 25 billion fat cells. Women have 68 percent more fat cells than men primarily because their bodies need to conceive and bear children. Extra fat offers a pregnant woman—under extreme conditions—more protection, warmth, and stored calories.

Approximately 90 percent of your fat cells were in place at your birth. Genetics plays a huge role in your future fatness or leanness. But, as a result of overeating, you can create new fat cells (approximately 10 percent). The primary times are during your first year, during puberty, and during pregnancy. Once you create new fat cells, they are yours for life. You can shrink them, but without surgery, you can't get rid of them.

Remember, shrinking fat is transferring fat—and transferring fat is effectively killing fat.

With the thermodynamics method involved in this book, you'll assume scientific management of your fat cells. You'll be able to stop obesity in its tracks; shrink the cells significantly; get rid of unwanted pounds and inches around your waist, hips, and thighs; rebuild your muscles; and strengthen your entire body.

What About Belly Bloat?

Belly bloat is often a female problem related to the menstrual cycle, hormonal changes, and water retention. Premenstrual syndrome, or PMS, is the term for a group of physical and mental symptoms that occur from five to eleven days before the beginning of a woman's menstrual cycle. PMS and belly bloat usually can be controlled by drinking plenty of water, cutting back on salt intake, and getting proper exercise and extra sleep. If the problem persists, aspirin, pain relievers, and regular use of birth control pills may be helpful.

There's another type of belly bloat that is not linked to hormones or the menstrual cycle. Both men and women can experience this type. The cause is gas trapped along the digestive tract, usually within the stomach and intestines. Gas comes from two main sources: swallowed air and the normal breakdown of certain foods by harmless bacteria naturally present in the digestive tract.

For many adults, too much gas can lead to a feeling of fullness and tightness along the front abdomen. Some of this gas may exit as flatulence. To deal effectively with this type of belly bloat requires application of some of the following practices.

How to Blast Belly Bloat

Steer Clear of Gas-Forming Foods: Certain foods contain sugars and starches that can be difficult for some people to digest. The most common culprits are legumes, such as lima beans, baked beans, and lentils. Other vegetables, such as broccoli, cauliflower, cabbage, Brussels sprouts, and turnips, can be problematic. Avoiding those foods is helpful. Sometimes, however, what it takes is consuming the problematic food for several days until your gastrointestinal tract has a chance to get better adapted, and then eating the foods more often.

Be Careful of Dairy Products and Lactose Intolerance: Many people have some form of lactose intolerance, which makes digesting dairy products difficult and results in gas. If your body can't break down lactose, eating most dairy products can result in bloating, constipation, or diarrhea. Remove dairy products from your diet for a week and see if your belly bloat is significantly reduced. There are also over-the-counter enzymes available that can be taken with lactose-containing foods to prevent these symptoms.

Reduce Salty (Sodium-Containing) Foods: If you consume more sodium than you need, your kidneys respond by holding on to extra water to keep the sodium content in your blood normal. Holding on to that extra water can make you feel inflated. Most chips, dips, and sauces—and many snack foods—are loaded with salt and sodium. One solution is to limit such foods and use low-sodium sauces in your recipes and at meals.

Drink More Water: Plenty of water is a curative for too much salt in your diet, and it can absolutely reduce belly bloat by simple dilution of the involved chemicals and gases. Be sure to study chapter 16 for all the latest guidelines on drinking more water each day. Equally important, you'll learn in chapter 16 how superhydration contributes to killing fat, building muscle, and overall health.

Slow Down Your Eating: Don't gulp down your food at a fast clip. Doing so automatically makes you swallow more air, which can swell your belly. Take your time. Put your fork on your plate after each bite. Try chewing each bite ten times or more before you swallow. You'll take in less air, and you'll probably eat fewer calories because you'll feel satiated sooner.

Stop Chewing Gum: Gum chewing can cause you to swallow more air, which can tend to balloon your belly. Plus, sugar-free gum, which is popular because of its lower calories, is sweetened with

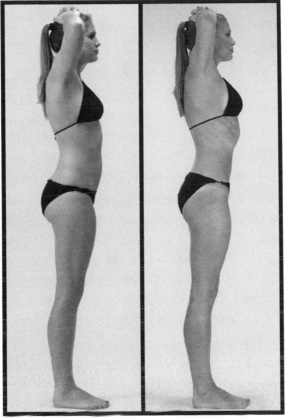

131.2 pounds   110.8 pounds

JENNIFER STANSFIELD, age 20, height 5'7"
AFTER 6 WEEKS
17.8 pounds of fat loss
4.6 inches off waist
6.4 pounds of muscle gain

substances that are only partially digestible. The partial-digestion process can cause gastrointestinal side effects including gas and bloating.

Beware of Carbonated Beverages: Cold carbonated drinks—such as colas, lemon-lime soda, and ginger ale—can certainly make you burp, which can be an effective way to get rid of excess air in your stomach. But some of what you consume doesn't get out with a burp. Instead, it leads to bloat. Sipping more plain water can help eliminate the distended feeling.

Lay Off the Alcohol: Beer, champagne, and some wines are carbonated, and also loaded with calories. Alcohol can produce bloating and negatively affect your digestion. Avoiding it is the best guideline.

Emphasize Foods Less Likely to Cause Gas: Included in this group are meat, poultry, fish, eggs, lettuce, tomatoes, zucchini, cantaloupe, berries, cherries, avocado, olives, and rice.

Keep Your Meals Small: One of the hallmarks of my Killing Fat eating plan is to consume smaller meals more often. A small meal is 300 calories for a woman and 400 calories for a man. Do not miss a meal and then try to make up for missing it by gorging yourself with twice as many calories at the next meal. Eat medium to small meals.

Catch Up on Your Sleep: A lot of adults tend to eat heavy at night and also squeeze in a midnight snack. My suggestion is to eat medium at night and have only a small late-night snack. With less digestion going on and no overstuffing, you'll sleep better, sounder, and longer.

Belly Bloat, Body Fat, and Thermodynamics

Belly bloat and body fat transferring on and off involve the cold-and-hot interplay of multiple chemicals within several systems. Controlling them requires an understanding of the science of thermodynamics.

With the thermodynamic synergy involved in this book, you'll be able to rein in belly bloat. You'll assume scientific management of your fat cells. You'll be prepared to shrink the cells significantly, get rid of unwanted pounds and inches, rebuild your muscles, and dramatically strengthen your entire body.

THE KILLING FAT FORMULA FOR SUCCESS

1 + 1 + 1 + 1 = 16

KILLING FAT WITH thermodynamics entails synergy. Synergy is the simultaneous occurrence of separate factors that together create greater total effect than the sum of their individual actions. By following the guidelines for successful fat transfer in chapter 1, you can expect your body to change drastically for the better—thanks to synergy. Yes, 1 + 1 + 1 + 1 in fat transfers will not = 4. It will equal 8, 10, or even 12 . . . and in only six to twelve weeks.

There's more.

As a benefit of my recently revealed secret, thermodynamic synergy, the total of 1 + 1 + 1 + 1 can equal 16. That's synergy with sizzle—a *lot* of sizzle!

Important: From a scientific (engineering) point of view, thermodynamic synergy cannot be a simple sum of equal factors. There must be some unknown synergistic factor that increases the additive value.

The real secret is recognition of the synergy among factors and the effect on the magnitude of the overall results. I don't think the actual numbers of the synergy are likely calculable. It is the teamwork of thermodynamic synergy and the overall fat loss that count. For example, in six weeks, a trainee loses 36.5 pounds of fat and drops 6 inches off his waist. Those results are measurable and photographable.

My latest Killing Fat program occurred in the fall of 2017. One interesting highlight involved three brothers.

The Sibling Fat-Loss Challenge

At twenty-seven years old, Noah Hastay was the youngest of the three brothers. Noah was the operations manager at Gainesville Health & Fitness and had worked there for five years. Because he was recovering from a back injury, Noah could not participate in the program. But he recruited his older brothers, Travis, 29, and Ian, 31, to join.

Both Travis and Ian had been basketball and soccer players in high school—and had suffered knee and ankle injuries that had required surgery and continued to bother them both. Plus, as with many athletes as they age, their appetites had gotten the best of them and they had gained significant fat: Travis had put on 60 pounds since he graduated from high school. Ian had gained even more, 77 pounds. They were willing and able to get started on my Killing Fat plan.

Two of the three brothers graduated from the University of Florida, and all were married, had families, and lived near Gainesville Health & Fitness—which made the action course more appealing to them.

I evaluated Travis's and Ian's initial condition and gave them some goals. My six-week challenge for the brothers was to drop a combined 83 pounds:

- **Travis:** Lose 43 pounds of fat.
- **Ian:** Lose 40 pounds of fat.

I wasn't disappointed: Travis lost 43.73 pounds of fat. Ian dropped 34.75. Combined, they lost a total of 78.48 pounds—just shy of my

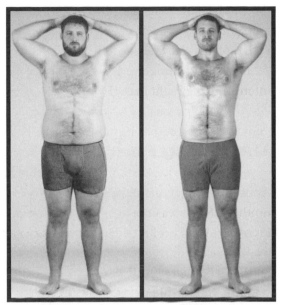

TRAVIS HASTAY,
age 29, height 6'4"
AFTER 12 WEEKS
58 pounds of fat loss
8.875 inches off waist
11.3 pounds of muscle gain

290.8 pounds   244 pounds

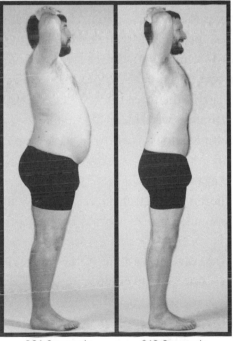

IAN HASTAY,
age 31, height 6'0"
AFTER 12 WEEKS
45.78 pounds of fat loss
8.375 inches off waist
4 pounds of muscle gain

261.6 pounds   219.8 pounds

83-pound challenge, but still enough to leave them in amazement. Plus, their waist reduction was right at 13 inches combined.

Travis and Ian decided to continue the program for six more weeks. At the completion of twelve weeks, Travis had lost 58 pounds of fat and Ian was down 45.78 pounds. That was a combined drop of almost 104 pounds of fat, which exceeded my goal for them by 21 pounds. Travis and Ian incorporated the Killing Fat formula for success. Travis was super strong, and it took a couple of workouts for him to get the 30–10–30 resistance just right, but when he did, the growth stimulation was full force and his muscles responded rapidly. Ian had some initial trouble with drinking a gallon of water each day, but soon he could feel the positive effects, which accelerated his results.

Brain Health and Stronger Muscles

When I was growing up in the 1950s and '60s, there was a common belief that if you lifted weights, you would become slow and muscle bound. Fortunately, the slow and muscle-bound concepts were dismissed by multiple research studies. By the year 2000, strength training was practiced by almost all sports teams—from high school through professional—in the United States.

It was proven repeatedly that bigger, stronger muscles made men and women better performers in all sports. It turns out that larger, stronger muscles may also be a key factor in protecting your brain and your memory.

Most men and women, once they get into their forties, begin losing muscle at the rate of approximately .5 pound per year. New research by Marnie Shaw from the Australia National University, published in the October 2017 edition of the *International Journal of Obesity*, reported that significant muscle atrophy can cause the brain's cortex to thin and shrink.

After testing 910 older subjects with magnetic resonance imaging (MRI) scans, Shaw and colleagues noted a pattern of cortical thinning in those people experiencing muscle loss, as opposed to those maintaining a stable body weight. These results suggest that losing muscle later in life is associated with brain changes that can increase the risk of dementia.

In another 2017 study, published in the journal *Alzheimer's & Dementia*, Mika Kivimaki and his team analyzed the association between body mass and brain health using data from more than 1.3 million adults from Europe, the United States, and Asia. Their report revealed that losing muscle mass, which is a common problem in older people, can be an early sign of dementia, twenty years before cognitive decline is noticeable.

Synergy in Action: Size Matters

Both of the 2017 studies concluded that it is important to stay strong and hold on to your muscle mass as long as possible. Your muscle power and brain health walk hand in hand throughout your life.

Doesn't it make sense that in the evolutionary history of humankind, the strongest men and strongest women would live the longest and reproduce the most? These two factors—strong muscles and active brains—have to be connected, understood, and applied with nutritious eating, superhydration, proper exercise, heat and cold transfer, and optimum recovery.

You are now in possession of the Killing Fat Formula for Success.

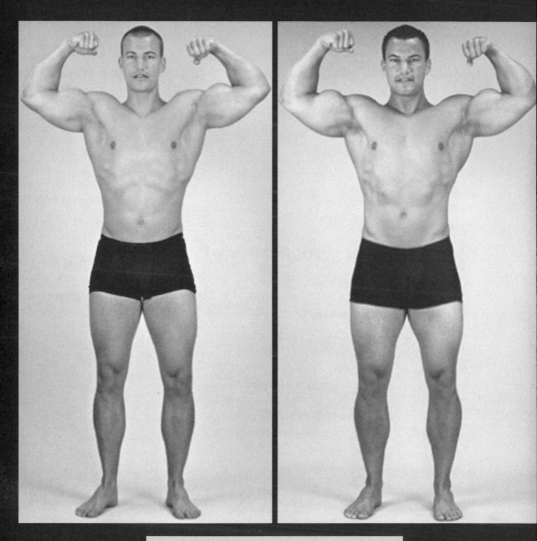

177 pounds   **194.25** pounds

JOE WALKER, age 26, height 5'9"
AFTER 6 WEEKS
(on muscle-building program only)
2 inches added on arms
2.5 inches added on chest
3 inches added on thighs
17.25 pounds of muscle gain

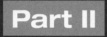
Part II

EATING AND EXERCISING FOR KILLING FAT

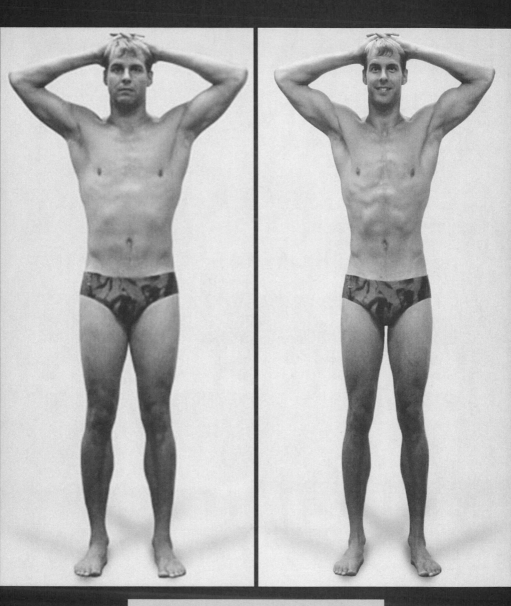

189.25 pounds   **171** pounds

GARY SMITH, age 29, height 6'1"
AFTER 6 WEEKS
20.5 pounds of fat loss
3.125 inches off waist
2.25 pounds of muscle gain

6

FOOD AND NUTRITION

THE NEW OLD-SCHOOL BASICS

I LEARNED BASIC NUTRITION in college courses in the 1960s and '70s. At that time, the emphasis was on eating a balanced diet

My eating concepts have changed somewhat since then, but you still need to be concerned with getting some forty-five nutrients almost every day. Nutrients fall into six classifications: carbohydrates, proteins, fats, vitamins, minerals, and water. Three of these groups—carbohydrates, proteins, and fats—contain calories or energy.

My balanced diet today applies the guidelines of the American Heart Association, which emphasize eating fat-free milk products, beans, fish, skinless poultry, and lean meats; using fats and oils with 2 grams or less of saturated fat per tablespoon; limiting foods high in calories or low in nutrition; eating fruits, vegetables, and whole-grain breads daily; and updating the weekly grocery list to include more green tea, garlic, and tomato-based condiments and sauces. Furthermore, I agree with the American Institute for Cancer Research's suggestion to maximize the intake of whole plant foods and minimize the intake of animal-based foods.

The Essential Nutrients

A *nutrient* is defined as a substance that supplies nourishment for growth and metabolism. In chapter 1, I noted that plants absorb nutrients primarily from the soil and animals obtain nutrients from foods they ingest (either plants or other animals that eat plants). Most people get their nutrients from the consumption of both plants and animals.

Throughout the twentieth century, nutritional scientists tested and retested a singular chemical or substance to determine if its absence would endanger health. Over many years, they have agreed that an adult requires forty-five essential nutrients. If you lack any one of the forty-five, sooner or later, your health will suffer.

The forty-five nutrients may be divided into the following:

- 19 minerals
- 13 vitamins
- 9 amino acids
- 2 fatty acids
- Glucose, a simple carbohydrate, for energy (calories)
- Water

The elements hydrogen, carbon, and nitrogen are not listed, as they are taken for granted as necessary from the environment. Oxygen is also essential, but nutritional science has traditionally limited itself to the study of nutrients that are absorbed by the body via the digestive system.

Food Groupings

Since 1894, the U.S. Department of Agriculture (USDA) has tried to figure out how to depict healthy-eating guidelines that would satisfy an individual getting all the essential nutrients. From 1943 to 1956, the guidelines were systematized into the "Basic Seven" food groups.

Dr. Fredrick Stare at Harvard University was instrumental in simplifying the Basic Seven into the "Basic Four" food groups, which I remember well from my third- and fourth-grade health classes. The Basic Four was used from 1956 to 1979, and included (1) Milk, (2) Meat, (3) Grain Products, and (4) Fruits and Vegetables. My nutrition professor at Florida State used the Basic Four in his lectures concerning nutrition and fat loss, and since then, I've applied the Basic Four formula successfully in many of my fat-loss programs.

From 1979 to 2011, the USDA expanded the Basic Four to five groups, then six, then a slightly different six, all arranged in a pyramid. Few people actually got the hang of the oddly shaped pyramid groupings, so there was thirty years of harsh criticism.

Finally, in 2011, the department simplified, condensed, and returned to four food groups (Protein, Grains, Fruits, and Vegetables) on a colorful plate, with a bit of Dairy on the side, which is in line with my own diet guidelines.

What About Sugar?

Nutritionally, there is virtually no difference among the various types of sugar.

In a typical manufacturing operation, sugarcane is shredded into small pieces and crushed, then processed to extract its juice. Further processing causes the juice to form sugar crystals and syrup, which are separated by a mechanical device into raw sugar and molasses. A washing-and-filtering process then turns the raw sugar into refined white sugar.

Real raw sugar cannot be sold in the United States because it contains contaminants, such as insect parts, soil, molds, bacteria, lint, and waxes. When partially refined to make it sanitary, it can be sold as "turbinado" sugar. Turbinado sugar is brown, but what we commonly call "brown sugar" is really refined white sugar coated with molasses (most manufacturers make it by spraying the molasses onto the sugar). Some people think turbinado and brown sugar look and smell more health-ful than white sugar. But the tiny amounts of additional nutrients they contain compared to refined white sugar are of no significance.

Fructose, a sugar present in fruits, is a little sweeter than sucrose. It may be slightly advantageous for use by some diabetics, but it is being widely promoted as healthier for everyone than sucrose—which it is not.

Honey is made from nectar gathered by bees. Depending on the source of the nectar, honey can vary slightly in composition and flavor. All honey is a blend of sugars, however, mostly fructose and glucose. Like brown sugar, honey contains tiny amounts of a few nu-trients. (An adult would have to consume 4 pounds of honey a day to get his Recommended Dietary Allowance of calcium, for example.) And there is no evidence that honey is easier to digest than other sug-ars. When you eat table sugar (sucrose), your body breaks it down into fructose and glucose—the two main sugars in honey.

A quick walk through a health food store may suggest that refined white sugar is rated on par with arsenic. But that does not mean sugar is eliminated in the products they sell. "Health" breads, for example, are full of honey, brown sugar, or raw sugar. Only refined white sugar is considered the villain.

It is true that many people consume too much sugar. But these same people also consume too many other carbohydrates, fats, and proteins, meaning that overall, they eat too many calories, which is one reason they are overweight.

There is no doubt that a sweet taste contributes to the pleasure of eating. Sugar, however, is neither better nor worse than many other foods. It is simply one component of a mixed diet.

Isn't Sugar Addictive?

In many people's minds, sugar must be addictive. They treat white sugar like many people did alcohol almost a century ago. But science notes there's a huge difference. Alcohol was and is a real addiction. Sugar is not.

According to the American Society of Addiction Medicine, addiction is a chronic disease of brain reward and related circuitry characterized by an inability to abstain consistently from the object of addiction. Cycles of relapse and remission are common, and without treatment, addiction is progressive and can lead to disability and even death.

For example, suddenly stopping a truly addictive drug, such as opioids and cocaine, will often cause side effects such as nausea, hot and cold flashes, anxiety, diarrhea, and insomnia.

Individuals who are denied a handful of Skittles, Nerds, or a chocolate bar don't experience those things. Instead, at worst, they get a bit crabby and cranky.

People also say that eating sugar lights up neural reward pathways just like certain drugs do. But scientists note that these same pathways also light up from playing video games, working out intensely, and sexual activity.

Furthermore, don't mistake ordinary cravings for true addiction— you sometimes desire a doughnut simply because you're responding to genetic blueprints laid down by your ancestors thousands of years ago. In pre-agricultural societies, food was, in general, not readily available. Thus, we were programmed to be attracted to the stuff (like sugar) that was high in calories and easy for the body to absorb.

What About Junk Foods?

Pizza, hamburgers, hot dogs, ice cream, candy, sodas, sugar, and potato chips have all individually been called "junk food." But think about that classification. Any food can be labeled "junk" if it is consumed excessively. That same food, if it is consumed in moderation with a correct variety of other foods, will not have a significant negative impact on your nutritional well-being.

What About All Those Chemicals in Processed Foods?

Chemicals are the building blocks of the natural world. You are made of chemicals, many different chemicals. In fact, according to the Mayo Clinic Libraries, the chemicals in your body, broken down into basic elements, are, in 2018, worth about $4.50. That's $3.50 for your skin and $1.00 for the rest of the oxygen, hydrogen, carbon, nitrogen, calcium, and phosphorus. Your deceased corpse would barely provide enough money for your relatives to purchase a nice orange at the supermarket. And interestingly, an average Valencia orange contains 219 chemicals, and many of them have long and scary-sounding names. In fact, if you were to break down almost any fruit or plant part into its chemical ingredients, you'd get a list that would look and sound menacing.

Advertisers tend to throw around words like "pure" and "simple" to describe "natural products," but they couldn't be more wrong. There's usually nothing simple about natural foods, but that isn't necessarily a bad thing, especially since Nature herself can construct things that, according to food scientist James Kennedy, are "far more complicated and unpredictable than anything we can produce in labs."

Stop bad-mouthing the long list of ingredients in the foods you buy. Just because you can't pronounce it doesn't mean it's harmful or bad. If that were the case, you'd never want to put soy sauce and wasabi on your sushi, and who would want to live in that kind of grim, gray world? We need man-made chemicals, and the difference between "natural" and "artificial" is often just a matter of perspective. After all, natural isn't always good for you, and the man-made stuff isn't always dangerous.

And what about processed foods—all those packaged, boxed, and canned products in your supermarket that have nutritional labels? According to some proponents of "eating clean," if a food's nutrition label lists more than one or two ingredients that you can't pronounce, do *not* put that food in your shopping basket.

If you adhere to that thinking, you'd never partake of a cup of plain coffee or tea. Coffee and tea contain dozens of scary-sounding chemicals.

Once again, how ridiculous.

Apply Your Intelligence

In the United States today, our supermarkets are stocked full of the most abundant, most nutritious, most economical, and safest supply of food that any people has ever had. The quality of this food was produced by the same precise, scientific processes that have given us other advances. Would the average American let anyone send us back to the days before automobiles, indoor flush toilets, or the internet? Of course not!

Remember the words of Carl Sagan in chapter 1:

If you don't use your intelligence, you risk becoming a fool.

. . . and Arthur Jones in the introduction:

Learn from your mistakes, move forward, and expand.

In chapter 7, I'll tell you how to plan and organize your Killing Fat eating plan for the best possible results. Not only do calories count, but carbohydrates do, too: carbs need to make up 50 percent of the total calories you consume per day.

Yes, it's time to say:

Welcome back, calories. Let's do some counting.

And welcome back, carbohydrates.

THE EATING PLAN

WELCOME BACK CARBOHYDRATES

ENTERED GRADUATE SCHOOL at Florida State University in Tallahassee in 1968 with all my strength-training beliefs about the fattening properties of carbohydrates and muscle-building effects of protein foods. Dr. Harold E. Schendel, my major nutrition professor at Florida State University from 1968 to 1973, was instrumental in switching my views and practices related to the importance of carbohydrates.

Schendel convinced me to experiment with my own body. A year of detailed study and critical analyses revealed that massive protein intakes did not work to my advantage in trying to build muscle and lose fat. In fact, I did not get the results I was after until I significantly lowered my protein intake and drastically increased my grams of carbohydrate each day.

I had been a reasonably successful competitive bodybuilder for ten years, so it was a difficult lesson for me to learn. But I did learn, and expand. In 1972, after two years of carbohydrate-rich eating, I finally won the bodybuilding title—Collegiate Mr. America—that I had chased for four years.

To Africa and Back

As I think back on my nutritional experiences at Florida State University, I remember vividly a story Schendel told me. In 1956, just having finished his PhD in nutritional biochemistry at the University of Illinois, he was hired by the University of Cape Town's medical school in South Africa. There he joined a team of doctors who were rushed into a drought-stricken area where a famine had been progressing for several years. Once organized, their initial objective was to assemble the starving children, who were suffering from kwashiorkor, and feed them a special high-protein diet.

After days of feeding—sometimes force-feeding—these bloated-bellied, tiny-limbed children, Schendel realized many of the children were getting worse and dying. "Why don't we try something different?" he asked. "Why don't we try a mush made with simple sugar, water, and butter?"

The new supplies were flown in and the mush was distributed. It worked. Force-feeding was no longer necessary. "The children loved the taste of the sugar, water, and butter," Schendel recalled. "The children lived . . . and began to stand and move around." After a week or so, Schendel and his team added small amounts of proteins, vitamins, and minerals to the mixture.

"I learned something of great value," Schendel remembered. "Starving bodies need calories in the form of simple sugars, simple carbohydrates. But many of my team, including me, had forgotten that. Thank God my nutritional studies on the importance of carbohydrates at Illinois were not in the distant past. Thank God for carbohydrates. Thank God for sugar."

I had been greatly influenced by reading muscle magazines and their cleverly designed collections of editorials, articles, and advertisements that promoted protein supplements and high-protein eating. Schendel reminded me repeatedly of the importance of carbohydrates in overall well-being.

During his four years in Africa, Schendel had saved many lives. In a way, he had also "saved" my life, because he and his eye-opening experiences had given me the motivation, ammunition, and energy to fight the bamboozle related to high-protein eating in both muscle building and fat loss.

Carbohydrate-rich eating is still doing that for me.

Hydrated Carbons and Protein Sparing

Another meaningful concept that I learned from Schendel related to the fact that humans have no way to capture solar energy. Plants, however, can and do, by using sunlight to combine carbon dioxide and water. The product of this combination is a hydrated carbon.

Look carefully at that term: *hydrated carbon*. Now turn it around: *car-bo-hy-drate*. Hydrated carbons and carbohydrates are one and the same. That's why carbohydrates in abundance are necessary to keep your body saturated with water. That's one reason carbohydrates saved the lives of many starving children in Africa: With carbohydrates in their systems, they could more easily hold on to what little water they could get.

Carbohydrates are also the body's preferred source of energy. And Schendel was always quick to point out to me—a bodybuilder—that carbohydrates were "protein sparing," meaning that adequate carbohydrates allow a moderate amount of dietary proteins to go a long way.

Said another way, the body can use proteins for energy, but it's a long process. It prefers to use carbohydrates for fast, sustainable energy.

What Schendel proved to me, and what is generally misunderstood by many fitness-minded individuals, was the following:

Carbohydrates should be emphasized, not neglected. The best sources of carbohydrates are vegetables, fruits, beans, and whole grains.

Don't be afraid to consume moderate amounts of sugar and refined-flour products.

Schendel believed that almost any food could be meaningful and healthy, with a little sugar thrown in for taste appeal.

A Look at the Basics

From my work with Dr. Schendel, the guidelines endorsed by the American Heart Association, the Academy of Nutrition and Dietetics (formerly the American Dietetic Association), my experiences with old-school nutrition, and my studies with thousands of fitness-minded people, I developed the following nutritional guidelines for losing fat:

- **Eat a diet high in complex carbohydrates.** Carbohydrates should comprise 50 percent or more of your total daily calories. Eat multiple servings of carbohydrates each day in the form of vegetables, fruits, whole grains, and legumes.
- **Sustain a moderate protein intake.** Protein should make up about 25 percent of your total daily calories if you are trying to lose fat. If you are trying to maintain your leanness, your protein can go down to 10 to 15 percent and carbohydrates can make up 60 to 65 percent. Choose low-fat sources of protein.
- **Maintain a total fat intake of 25 percent of your daily calories.** Limit your intake of fat by selecting lean meats, poultry without skin, fish, and low-fat dairy products. In addition, cut back on vegetable oils and butter—or foods made with these—as well as mayonnaise, salad dressings, and fried foods.
- **Avoid too much sugar.** Many foods that are high in sugar are also high in fat. Note that I did *not* say "No white sugar (sucrose)." White sugar in small amounts not only improves the taste of many foods, but it is acceptable on my eating plan.
- **Don't drink alcohol.** Alcoholic beverages can add many calories to your diet without supplying other nutrients. And excessive alcohol consumption can lead to a variety of health problems.
- **Drink more water, plain and cold.**

Calories per Day

In spite of what some popular authors would have you believe, the laws of thermodynamics are constant. All things in nature—including human metabolism—are governed by thermodynamics.

One gram of carbohydrate and 1 gram of protein each contain 4 calories, while 1 gram of fat contains 9 calories. All calories from carbohydrates, proteins, and fats count toward the surplus, or deficit, of fat metabolism. Once it is consumed, there is no way to weaken, discount, or bypass a food's calories. To lose fat, you must consume fewer calories than you burn each day.

Your calories per day should not be too low, or your body may pull nutrients from your muscles and vital organs, which is not desirable. The majority of people I've worked with achieve optimum fat-loss results by adhering to daily calorie levels that range from 1,800 to 1,400 for men, depending on body size, and 1,500 to 1,200 for women.

During my six-week Killing Fat program, I like to decrease daily calories by 100 with each two-week period. Such a gradual reduction makes your body more efficient at the fat-burning process. My recommended calories per day for the six-week program are as follows:

Men: 1,600 (weeks 1 and 2), 1,500 (weeks 3 and 4), and 1,400 (weeks 5 and 6)

Women: 1,400 (weeks 1 and 2), 1,300 (weeks 3 and 4), and 1,200 (weeks 5 and 6)

Meal Size

Fat loss is aided by eating small meals. There's a thin line between a small meal and a medium meal. I draw that line at 400 calories for women and 500 calories for men.

A large meal, or a meal of 1,000 calories or more (typical in the United States), triggers excessive insulin production. Insulin is your body's most powerful pro-fat hormone. Small meals of 400 calories or fewer bring on small insulin responses. Thus, it is to your advantage to consume downsized meals.

Meal Frequency

The goal is six small, evenly spaced meals a day. "Evenly spaced" means no longer than three hours should elapse between each eating episode: breakfast, lunch, and dinner; and snacks at midmorning, midafternoon, and night. In this book, a snack consisting of 100 to 200 calories counts as one of your six meals. Meals over 200 calories are reserved for breakfast, lunch, and dinner.

The size of your six meals, the time between them, and the total number of calories you consume each day have all been calculated and assembled for your convenience in chapter 11.

DR. KEN SPALDING: CARBOHYDRATES AND CONSISTENCY

From 2011 through 2018, I strength-trained Dr. Ken Spalding 264 times. When I met Ken, he was soft-spoken and told me up front that he didn't like heavy leg work. But at the same time, he wanted me to push him hard on his leg exercises, which I have done. Interestingly, Ken has only had one not-up-to-par workout in seven years—which is quite an achievement.

Ken's work ethic is also strong in his medical career. Several of his colleagues have noted to me that Dr. Spalding is the number one anesthesiologist at Florida Hospital in Orlando, especially in pediatrics.

I've noticed many times how vigilant Ken is in his meal planning and eating. Let him take you inside his experience with the Killing Fat program:

> I was first introduced to the writings of Dr. Ellington Darden in 1988, when I was a college student in Baltimore. At the time, I was working as an instructor at a Nautilus Fitness Center, and The Nautilus Book was required reading.
>
> After medical school at the University of Maryland, I did my pediatrics and anesthesiology residencies at the University of Florida College of Medicine. During residency, I was a member of Gainesville Health & Fitness, where Dr. Darden was doing research. One of his books, Living Longer Stronger, became the blueprint for how I have approached strength training and eating.
>
> In 2011, I heard that Dr. Darden lived a few miles from my home in Orlando, Florida. I visited him and joined his Intensive Coaching program, in which I have continued to train for seven years.

THE IMPORTANCE OF CARBOHYDRATES

I've had a longtime interest in nutrition and have followed the diet industry closely. I was intrigued by the popular low-carbohydrate plans. I tried many of them and, in fact, lost weight. Like many people, however, I just couldn't stick with this diet long term.

What must be kept in mind is that all diets, whether low-carbohydrate or not, have one thing in common: They are all calorie-restricted. As Dr. Darden has pointed out in this and earlier chapters, the laws of thermodynamics are always in effect.

To lose fat, fewer calories must be consumed than are expended. It's true that some individuals following a low-carbohydrate diet tend to lose weight more quickly than those on a calorie-restricted diet. This can be explained by a greater initial loss of body fluids, and the tendency of people on low-carbohydrate diets to eat less.

The belief that there is some metabolic advantage for fat loss on a low-carbohydrate diet remains unproven. What is known is that the initial weight loss advantage of a low-carbohydrate diet wanes as time progresses. Low-carbohydrate diets are not sustainable in the long term. An eating plan containing 50 to 60 percent of calories from carbohydrates can be used to achieve a person's desired weight and be modified by adding or subtracting calories as needed.

CONSISTENCY A MUST

What is the key to remaining lean and fit into my fifties? I can sum it up in one word: *CONSISTENCY.*

Day after day, week after week, month after month—you must be steady, dependable, and unfailing in your actions and practices.

With Dr. Darden's books, I've found an overall fitness plan that works, and I believe I can follow it for life. Most important, I believe the plan can be adapted for almost anyone. Here are my guidelines:

- Weigh yourself regularly.
- Discern a trigger weight that prompts a reevaluation and a correction of eating habits (for me, that's 172 pounds).
- Adopt an eating plan that allows you to make the correction.
- Keep your carbohydrates at 50 percent of total calories.
- Use a high-intensity strength-training routine twice a week.
- Do a cardio-aerobic activity several times a week.
- Stay well hydrated and rest adequately.

Remember: Consistency is the key to getting the fat off *and* the key to keeping it off.

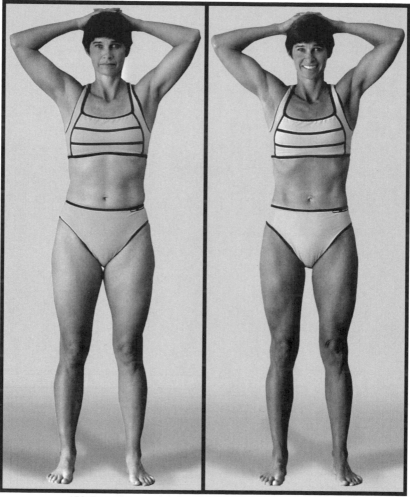

150.5 pounds   **134.25** pounds

JANE KNUTH, age 40, height 5'9"
AFTER 6 WEEKS
19.25 pounds of fat loss
2.875 inches off waist, **4.25** inches off thighs
3 pounds of muscle gain

8

THE BEST TYPE OF EXERCISE FOR FAT LOSS

NEGATIVE-ACCENTUATED TRAINING

THE VARIOUS SKELETAL muscles of your body have the ability to contract or shorten, and to hold and support weight. But these muscles also have the capacity to lengthen, stretch, and—although it's not the correct term—*uncontract*.

Physiologists have named the contraction process concentric muscle action. The lengthening maneuver is called eccentric muscle action. In these contexts, *concentric* means moving toward the center of the body and *eccentric* means moving away from the center.

I've mentioned this earlier, but as a quick review: An exercise to use as an example would be the standing biceps curl with a barbell. Stand holding a moderately heavy barbell and smoothly curl the bar up to your shoulders. Then slowly lower it down to your thighs. The up movement involves concentric action of the biceps muscles. The down, or lowering, movement requires eccentric muscle action of the same muscles of the biceps.

Bodybuilders, weight lifters, and strength coaches simplify concentric and eccentric muscle actions by using the words *positive* (concentric) and *negative* (eccentric). In strength-training circles, lifting a weight is positive and lowering it is negative. The same is true of a weight machine: As the weight stack moves up, positive work is performed. As it moves down, negative work is accomplished.

For ease of understanding, especially for the recommended exercises involved in this book, I'll use the words *positive* and *negative* instead of *concentric* and *eccentric*.

For more than sixty-five years, researchers have compared the various aspects of positive and negative work. In 1953, Erling Asmussen, PhD, an exercise physiologist at the University of Copenhagen, Denmark, was the first to point out in a scientific journal the differences between positive and negative work, though the measuring tools and techniques he applied were crude. In the 1980s, thanks to my colleague Arthur Jones of Nautilus Sports/Medical Industries, the tools and techniques became more valid and the results repeatable.

Jones discovered that both women and men were approximately 40 percent stronger in the negative stroke of an exercise machine compared to the positive stroke. Jones's research opened the door for athletes and fitness-minded people to apply negative work in their weekly strength-training programs. But because of the precision of techniques involved, and the probability of misunderstanding, both scientific and lay publications over the last twenty-five years were riddled with little consistency and scattered results.

Marc Roig and His Work

Marc Roig, PhD, in 2008, was head of the Muscle Biophysics Laboratory at the University of British Columbia in Vancouver. Roig and his colleagues saw the disparities in the published research and decided to sort things out by using newer types of statistical tests called meta-analyses. Meta-analysis comprises statistical methods for contrasting and combining findings from individual studies in the quest to identify patterns among their results.

Roig's group carefully examined all the studies published over the last fifty years that compared negative-style resistance training with normal positive training. At first, they identified 1,954 titles from their literature search. Of this number, 276 were suitable for abstract review. More than sixty publications made the next cut. Deeper examinations, such as poor directions in testing and potential crossover effect, narrowed the studies down to exactly twenty.

These twenty studies involved a total of 678 subjects. The usual training frequency was three times per week and the duration of the experiments ranged from four to twenty-five weeks, with the most popular duration being six weeks. Entering all the data from those studies, the computerized meta-analyses, as reported in 2009 in the *British Journal of Sports Medicine*, revealed the following:

Negative training was significantly more effective in increasing muscular size and strength than positive-style training.

Roig's report was published online on November 3, 2008, and I remember reading it with much interest. Not only had I been interested in negative training for more than twenty years, but in early October 2008, I had been contacted by Mats Thulin of Stockholm, Sweden, who told me he had successfully designed a machine that accentuated the negative.

Mats Thulin and X-Force

I flew to Stockholm on November 13, 2008, to meet with Thulin and try his new negative-accentuated equipment. Thulin called his machines X-Force, and they operated differently from any other type of exercise equipment I'd ever seen.

The approach Thulin applied involves a tilting weight stack powered by an electric servomotor. As the user begins the positive stroke, the weight stack is at a 45-degree angle. This angle reduces the selected resistance significantly. At the top of the positive stroke, the tilted weight stack returns to vertical and the resistance is instantly 40 percent heavier. The user then lowers 100 percent of the selected resistance.

After training with X-Force for three days and discussing the parameters and physiology with Thulin and his team, I was convinced of its overall potential. The ingenuity of the X-Force equipment is a patented, tilting weight stack that unloads the positive phase and then overloads the negative. X-Force's fourteen strength-training machines supply negative-accentuated exercise—40 percent extra negative resistance compared to the positive—without the use of assistants.

When I returned to the United States, I knew I had to get a line of X-Force machines installed in Florida so I could continue my progression in better ways to lose fat and build muscle. One of the first people I talked with about X-Force was Joe Cirulli of Gainesville Health & Fitness. Cirulli and I had pursued various fat-loss and muscle-building projects together over the years, and X-Force was no exception.

It took a lot of discussion and planning, but in January 2012, Cirulli's club was outfitted with fourteen X-Force machines. Gainesville and Orlando are an easy drive from each other, so I knew I could quickly get a research project together. Thus, on February 6, 2012, I started my first group training on X-Force equipment. By December 2012, I had trained eight groups on X-Force, with a total of 145 participants from Gainesville Health & Fitness. The research experiences, data, and photographs were combined into a book, *The Body Fat Breakthrough: Tap the Muscle-Building Power of Negative Training and Lose Up to 30 Pounds in 30 Days*.

Basically, the X-Force program in Gainesville that worked so well involved performing one set of 6 to 8 repetitions on each of six machines, with each repetition done to a count of a 3-second positive, immediately followed by a 5-second negative. Any time a trainee did 8 or more repetitions correctly, the resistance was increased by 5 percent at the next workout. The frequency of the workouts was twice a week.

Halfway through the book project, I realized I needed an alternative method of exercising for people who don't have access to X-Force. In *The Body Fat Breakthrough*, that alternative method is called 30–30–30.

30–30–30

Through trial-and-error testing, 30–30–30 proved to be a results-producing alternative to X-Force. In Gainesville, I trained a dozen or so people in this manner, with excellent results.

To perform 30–30–30 properly, take 80 percent of the resistance you'd normally handle for 10 repetitions with a barbell or weight machine. Have an assistant help you get the resistance to the top position. Then do a slow 30-second negative, followed by a 30-second positive, followed by a final 30-second negative. That's 1.5 repetitions, or 60 seconds of negative work and 30 seconds of positive work. That's one set, and that's all you need to do for each of six exercises. The exercises I selected were the leg press, leg curl, leg extension, chest press, lat pulldown to chest, overhead press, curl, and abdominal crunch.

While 30–30–30 proved to be a very good way to strengthen and build muscle, it was also difficult for people to get the hang of. Many trainees simply said, "30–30–30 is too hard. I don't enjoy exercising in this fashion."

So I decided to experiment with some variations of this slow method to see if I could discover a style that was slightly less intense but equally productive. Remember, I still wanted to accentuate the negative, because I knew the negative phase offered the most benefits.

After a couple of months of experimentation, I came up with what I call 15–15–15, plus 8 to 12 repetitions. Instead of taking 30 seconds to perform a slow negative, each phase was shortened to 15 seconds. Compared to 30–30–30, this new technique was somewhat easier, which proved to be a nice alternative, especially for women.

In the 15–15–15 method, you take 80 percent of what you'd normally handle on a resistance exercise. Get the barbell or resistance mechanism to the top position quickly, then do a 15-second negative, followed by a 15-second positive, then a 15-second negative. But don't stop there—continue doing a series of faster, complete repetitions to a count of approximately 1 second on the positive and 2 seconds on the negative. Your goal is 8 to 12 of these faster repetitions. And again, only one set each of these six to eight exercises is necessary, which are practiced twice a week.

15–15–15 worked well on short-range abdominal floor exercises, body-weight movements such as the squat and push-up, and dumbbell exercises such as the curl and overhead press. But I still was not satisfied. I needed a technique that involved a bit more "punch." That's when I came up with a hybrid of 30–30–30 and 15–15–15, plus 8 to 12. I called this new method 30–10–30.

30–10–30: A Hybrid with a Punch

In chapter 3, I gave you a preview of a barbell curl in the 30–10–30 style. Basically, what you have is a slow 30-second negative repetition, which certainly tires the involved muscles. Immediately, with the same resistance, you perform 10 normal repetitions, taking approximately 1 second on the positive and 2 seconds on the negative. Now your biceps are fatigued significantly, but that's not all. With the barbell still in the top position of the curl, you make a final attempt at a 30-second negative. What you have is a 30-second negative repetition, 10 faster positive-negative repetitions, and a final 30-second negative repetition—thus the name: 30–10–30.

But, and this is important, the name 30–10–30 involves more than those meaningful numbers. In practice, the 30-second negatives can vary from 15 to 30 seconds. Frequently, a trainee can manage the first negative repetition in 30 seconds but can barely get 15 seconds on the finishing negative. Thus, on his workout sheet, his notation would read "30–10–15." Or sometimes, both the first and second negative might be a little fast, so the notation might read "25–10–25."

Then, in actual high-intensity training, the faster middle repetitions are not always 10. Sometimes, you can only do 7, 8, or 9, so your record might read "30–8–30." Or on a great training day, you might do an easy 10 repetitions and need to do two more to get the right feel, for "30–12–30."

The idea is always to work to momentary muscular fatigue, especially on the in-between positive-negative repetitions and the finishing negative.

When you can complete any exercise in 30–12–30, that is the signal to increase the resistance by 3 to 5 percent for your next workout.

The next chapter will provide you with all the details and illustrations on how to plan and perform 30–10–30 routines with the recommended exercises.

9

THE 30–10–30 EXERCISES

FREE WEIGHTS AND MACHINES

THIS CHAPTER FEATURES eighteen recommended exercises: ten with free weights and eight with machines. All the basic movements for the major muscles of your body are covered and illustrated.

Since 2015, I've tried and tested the exercises in this chapter with twenty-one of my Intensive Coaching trainees here in Orlando. I put a team of twelve firemen through a six-week program of 30–10–30 exercises in 2016. A group of eight young men from Gainesville Health & Fitness attacked the exercises with enthusiasm in the fall of 2017. Finally, my longtime friend Jim Flanagan—who has a home gym of Nautilus and MedX strength-training equipment in Longwood, Florida, 25 miles from where I live—has applied 30–10–30 successfully with eight of his trainees, including himself.

"I really like 30–10–30," Flanagan noted. "It makes you slow down and practice precision form. Plus, the gains are outstanding. It's now a permanent part of my high-intensity training techniques."

In the last three years, forty-nine individuals have been trained intensely during multiple workouts using my 30–10–30 method. As a result, I've been able to give each exercise a thorough examination, and you'll receive my best instruction on how to get the full benefits from each one.

Get Ready to Focus

On the remaining pages of this chapter, you'll find my recommended exercises for the 30–10–30 method of negative-accentuated training. Each movement is illustrated and the steps outlined under the following headings:

Preparation: Equipment required and starting position

First Negative: A description of the lowering phase of the movement

Regular Reps: An explanation of how to do the normal positive-negative reps

Finish Negative: A description of the final negative part of the exercise and how to make it more effective

Tips: Details to improve the results

For most of the photos in this chapter, image A indicates the starting position of the negative, and image B is the starting point of the regular positive-negative reps.

Important note: To standardize the guidelines, all the 30-second negatives will be described applying 20 seconds. I do this because it's a great way to start. After you become familiar with the technique and build more strength, you will progress to 25-second negatives and, finally, to the ideal 30-second negatives. As a result, the illustrated exercises will be described as "20–10–20." That is a 20-second negative, 10 normal-speed positive-negative reps, followed by a final 20-second negative.

FREE-WEIGHT NEGATIVES

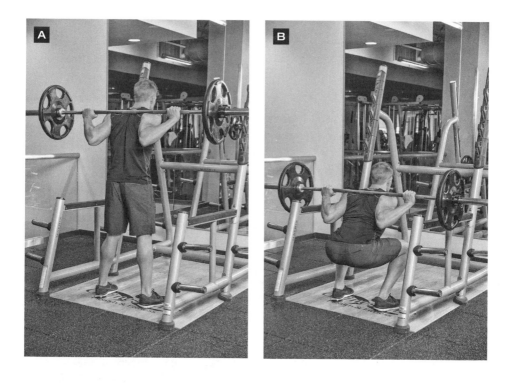

BARBELL SQUAT

MUSCLES WORKED: Gluteus maximus, quadriceps, hamstrings, and erector spinae

PREPARATION
- Have a watch with a second hand—or, better yet, a big clock with a second hand—in plain sight, or have a spotter help with the counting.
- Place a barbell inside a power rack in the top position on the hooks. Or use squat racks similar to the above photos.

- Take two horizontal restraint bars and place them appropriately in the lowest deep-squat position of your range of motion. (These bars protect you from going too low, losing your balance, and possibly injuring yourself.)
- Load the barbell with the appropriate amount of resistance.
- Position the bar behind your neck across your trapezius muscles and hold the bar in place with your hands. If the bar cuts into your skin, pad it lightly by wrapping a towel around the knurl.
- Straighten your knees to lift the bar from the hooks and move back one step.
- Place your feet shoulder-width apart, toes angled slightly outward. Keep your upper-body muscles rigid and your torso upright during this exercise.

FIRST NEGATIVE
- Bend your hips and knees slowly, inch by inch.
- Descend gradually to the half-squat position in 10 seconds.
- Squat a little farther to three-quarters level.
- Reach the bottom position, in which your hamstrings firmly come in contact with your calves, in 20 seconds.
- Make the turnaround gradually from negative to positive and get ready to begin the regular reps.

REGULAR REPS
- Perform 10 barbell squats smoothly at a speed of 1 second for the positive and 2 seconds for the negative. Push yourself to complete 10 repetitions, but remember, the regular repetitions may vary between 8 and 12. The idea is to do as many as you can in good form.
- After your last rep, get ready for the finish negative.

FINISH NEGATIVE
- Bend your hips and knees smoothly and slowly.
- Hit the halfway-down mark at 10 seconds and the three-quarters mark at 15 seconds.

- Keep your focus and continue breathing freely.
- Hold the resistance off the bottom restraint bars, in the deep-squat position, for a final second or two.
- Transfer the barbell to the bottom restraint bars. Sit down on the floor, or stagger out of the power rack carefully, and relax.

TIPS

- Do not allow your torso to bend forward on the positive reps of the squat. Doing so takes some of the force off your thighs and places it on your lower back, which can be dangerous.
- As a safety measure, it's also a good idea to use one or two spotters during the barbell squat.

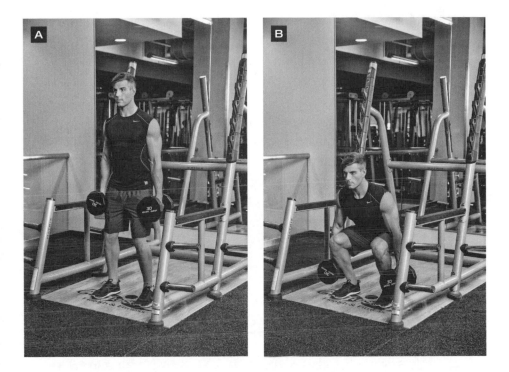

DUMBBELL SQUAT

MUSCLES WORKED: Gluteus maximus, quadriceps, hamstrings, and erector spinae

PREPARATION

- Have a watch with a second hand—or, better yet, a big clock with a second hand—in plain sight, or have a spotter help with the counting.
- Grasp a dumbbell in each hand and stand. The dumbbells should be hanging down by the outsides of your thighs.
- Place your feet a little wider than shoulder-width apart, with your toes angled out slightly.
- Keep your upper-body muscles rigid, chest out, and torso upright.

FIRST NEGATIVE

- Start bending your knees slightly, inch by inch.
- Push your hips and butt back as if you were going to close a door behind you with your butt. Keep a slight arch in your lower back.
- Reach the half-squat position at the 10-second mark.
- Squat a little lower to the three-quarters level. Keep your heels on the floor. The dumbbells should now be hanging comfortably near the outsides of your calves.
- Be at your lowest level at 20 seconds. Go as low as you can without lifting your heels. The dumbbells should almost touch the floor.
- Push down through your heels, not your toes, and get ready to begin the regular reps.

REGULAR REPS

- Perform 10 dumbbell squats smoothly at a speed of 1 second for the positive and 2 seconds for the negative. Push yourself to complete 10 repetitions, but remember, the regular repetitions may vary between 8 and 12. The idea is to do as many as you can in good form.
- Keep breathing, with your chest high. Do not hold your breath.
- After your last rep, get ready for the finish negative.

FINISH NEGATIVE

- Repeat the slow lowering, inch by inch.
- Focus, breathe, and keep your torso rigid.
- Try to keep your arms relaxed. Use them as hangers, with the dumbbells at the end.
- Be halfway down at 10 seconds. The hardest part is from halfway down to the bottom.
- Place the dumbbells on the floor at 20 seconds. Stand and relax your thighs.

TIPS

- Note that your shape and flexibility can affect how deeply you can squat with the dumbbells. Some people have difficulty squatting below a level where the tops of their thighs are parallel to the floor. Others can almost touch their buttocks to their heels.
- If your ankles are tight and you tend to lift your heels at the bottom of the squat, try placing a 1-inch-thick board under your heels for stability.

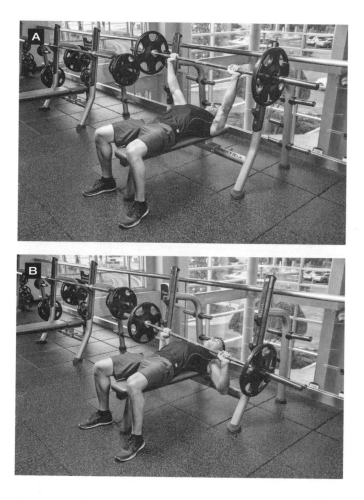

BARBELL BENCH PRESS

MUSCLES WORKED: Pectoralis major, deltoids, and triceps

PREPARATION

- Have a watch with a second hand—or, better yet, a big clock with a second hand—in plain sight, or have a spotter help with the counting.

- Set up a barbell with an appropriate resistance on the support racks of a flat bench.
- Lie on your back on the bench.
- Grasp the barbell with your hands positioned slightly more than shoulder-width apart.
- Straighten your arms and bring the barbell to a supported position above your sternum.

FIRST NEGATIVE
- Lower the barbell slowly, inch by inch.
- Try to be halfway down at 10 seconds and three-quarters down at 15 seconds.
- Touch your sternum at 20 seconds, but do not rest.
- Make a smooth turnaround and get ready to begin the regular reps.

REGULAR REPS
- Press the barbell to full extension in approximately 1 second.
- Lower the bar smoothly in approximately 2 seconds. Again, that's a 1-second positive and a 2-second negative.
- Make the bottom and top turnarounds under control and continue for 10 repetitions.
- Keep the movements steady. Do not rest.
- Stop at the top of the tenth repetition and get ready for the finish negative.

FINISH NEGATIVE
- Control the negative and lower the bar inch by inch.
- Be halfway down at 10 seconds.
- Fight the lowering. Don't let the resistance force the bar downward too fast.
- Reach the bottom at 20 seconds.

- Have the spotter quickly help you get the barbell back to the support racks at the top.
- Move off the bench and relax.

TIPS

- This exercise takes some practice. During your first workout, play it safe and use only 60 percent of the weight you'd normally handle for 10 repetitions.
- Stabilize your starting position by squeezing your shoulder blades together and holding them that way throughout the exercise. Make sure the bar remains directly above your elbows at all times.
- Avoid using a wide grip on the bench press. Since the function of your pectoral muscles is to move your upper arms across your torso, spacing your hands wider than your shoulders actually shortens your range of motion. Rather than working more of your chest muscles, you're working fewer of them.
- Use a spotter on the barbell bench press.

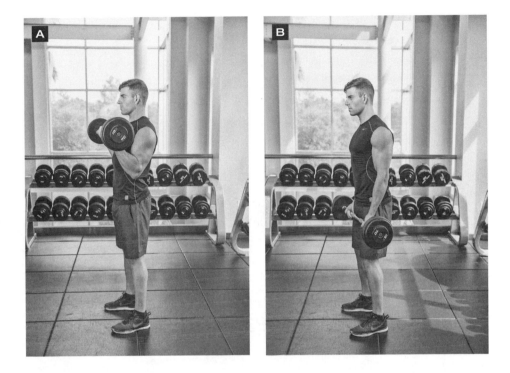

BARBELL CURL

MUSCLES WORKED: Biceps of upper arms

PREPARATION

- Have a watch with a second hand—or, better yet, a big clock with a second hand—in plain sight, or have a spotter help with the counting.
- Take a shoulder-width underhand grip on the barbell. As you stand with the barbell, use some upward momentum and curl the weight efficiently to your shoulders.
- Anchor your elbows firmly against your sides and get ready for the first negative.

FIRST NEGATIVE

- Lower the weight gradually, inch by inch.
- Reach the halfway-down position at 10 seconds, and do not move your elbows backward. Anchor them against your sides for the entire lowering.
- Keep your torso erect as you near the bottom at 20 seconds.
- Get ready to begin the regular reps.

REGULAR REPS

- Curl the weight in approximately 1 second to your shoulders.
- Lower the bar smoothly in approximately 2 seconds. Again, that's a 1-second positive and a 2-second negative.
- Make the bottom and top turnarounds under control and continue for 10 repetitions.
- Keep the movements steady. Do not rest.
- Stop at the top of the tenth repetition and get ready for the finish negative.

FINISH NEGATIVE

- Control the negative and lower the bar inch by inch.
- Be halfway down at 10 seconds.
- Unbend your arms and be near the bottom at 20 seconds.
- Keep holding the bar with your biceps until the count is 20.
- Place the barbell on the floor and relax.

TIP

- Maximize your biceps stimulation by minimizing your body sway: Do not lean forward excessively or lean backward. Do not move your upper arms. Do not move your head. Move only your hands, your forearms, and the barbell.

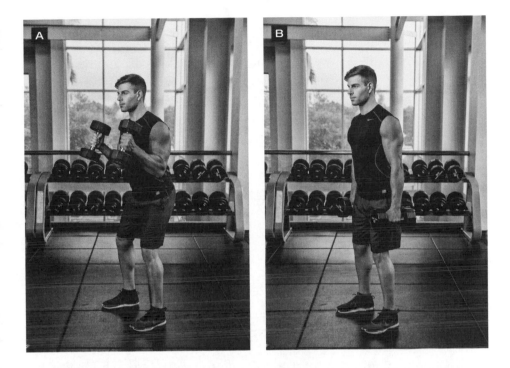

DUMBBELL HAMMER CURL

MUSCLES WORKED: Brachialis, biceps, and brachioradialis

PREPARATION

- Have a watch with a second hand—or, better yet, a big clock with a second hand—in plain sight, or have a spotter help with the counting.
- Grasp a dumbbell in each hand and stand with your feet shoulder-width apart.
- Turn the dumbbells so your palms are facing your torso, similar to the way you'd hold a hammer.
- Use some upward momentum and curl the dumbbells to your shoulders.
- Anchor your elbows firmly against your sides and get ready to begin the first negative.

FIRST NEGATIVE

- Lower the dumbbells together slowly, inch by inch.
- Reach the halfway-down position at 10 seconds, and do not move your elbows backward. Anchor them against your sides for the entire lowering and continue holding the dumbbells hammer-style.
- Keep your torso erect as you near the bottom at 20 seconds.
- Get ready to begin the regular reps.

REGULAR REPS

- Curl the dumbbells hammer style in approximately 1 second to your shoulders.
- Lower the dumbbells smoothly in approximately 2 seconds. Again, that's a 1-second positive and a 2-second negative.
- Make the bottom and top turnarounds under control and continue for 10 repetitions.
- Keep the movements steady. Do not rest.
- Stop at the top of the tenth repetition and get ready to begin the finish negative.

FINISH NEGATIVE

- Lower the dumbbells inch by inch.
- Be halfway down at 10 seconds.
- Unbend your arms and be near the bottom at 20 seconds.
- Keep holding the dumbbells with your brachialis and biceps until the count is 20.
- Place the dumbbells on the floor and relax.

TIP

- Maximize your brachialis and biceps stimulation by minimizing your body sway: Do not lean forward excessively or lean backward. Do not move your upper arms. Do not move your head. Move only your hands, your forearms, and the dumbbells.

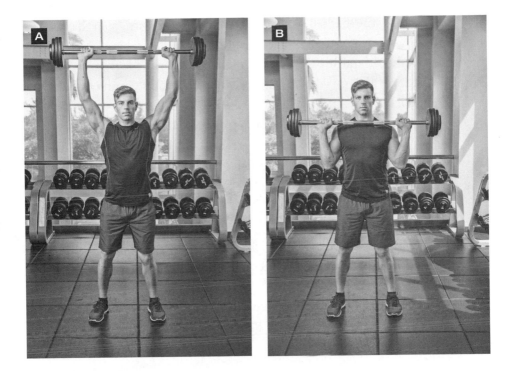

BARBELL OVERHEAD PRESS

MUSCLES WORKED: Deltoids and triceps

NOTE
Even with a 50-pound barbell, this is a tough, challenging exercise. Be careful.

PREPARATION
- Have a watch with a second hand—or, better yet, a big clock with a second hand—in plain sight, or have a spotter help with the counting.
- Place a barbell in a power rack on mid-chest-high hooks.
- Load the bar with an appropriate amount of weight.

- Grasp the barbell with an overhand grip with your hands slightly wider than shoulder-width apart.
- Unhook and lift the barbell, mostly with your legs, and step back with it on your shoulders. Make sure your feet and legs are in a stable position.
- Bend your knees slightly and push press the barbell overhead. With your elbows completely straight, the barbell should be directly above your shoulders. Get ready to begin for the negative phase, as you'll be lowering the bar to your shoulders.

FIRST NEGATIVE

- Lower the barbell slowly, inch by inch.
- Be halfway down at 10 seconds and three-quarters down at 15 seconds.
- Focus on your breathing, especially quick exhalations.
- Touch your upper chest at 20 seconds and turn the movement around to begin the regular reps.

REGULAR REPS

- Begin your regular-speed barbell presses smoothly, taking 1 second for the positive and 2 seconds for the negative.
- Try to complete 10 repetitions.
- Stop at the top of the tenth repetition and get ready to begin the finish negative.

FINISH NEGATIVE

- Lower the barbell slowly, inch by inch.
- Be halfway down at 10 seconds and three-quarters down at 15 seconds.
- Try to control the movement by breathing out at a rapid rate.
- Touch the bar to your upper chest at 20 seconds.
- Move back carefully to the power rack and place the bar securely on the hooks.
- Exit the power rack and relax.

TIPS

- Keep your lower back naturally arched during the movements.
- The negative-accentuated overhead press is an excellent exercise for your shoulders and arms, although it can be somewhat challenging for both women and men. It may take you several practice sessions to learn the mechanics of it.

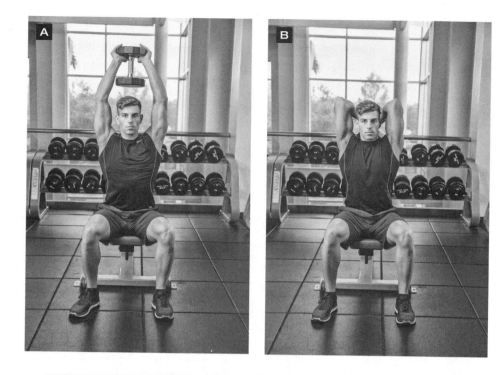

DUMBBELL TRICEPS EXTENSION

MUSCLES WORKED: Triceps

PREPARATION

- Have a watch with a second hand—or, better yet, a big clock with a second hand—in plain sight, or have a spotter help with the counting.
- Sit on a bench. Grasp a dumbbell at one end with both hands.
- Extend the dumbbell overhead.
- Pull your elbows in tight and keep them close to your ears throughout the exercise, and get ready to begin the first negative.

FIRST NEGATIVE

- Bend your elbows and lower the dumbbell slowly, inch by inch.
- Reach the halfway-down position at 10 seconds.

- Be careful not to move your elbows. Only your forearms and hands should move.
- Reach the bottom position, with the dumbbell behind your neck, at 20 seconds.
- Get ready to begin the regular reps.

REGULAR REPS

- Extend the dumbbell smoothly overhead in 1 second and immediately lower it in 2 seconds.
- Do 10 repetitions in good form.
- Stop at the top of the tenth repetition and get ready to begin the finish negative.

FINISH NEGATIVE

- Repeat the procedures on the first negative.
- Be halfway down at 10 seconds.
- Focus and keep good form. Relax your face and breathe.
- Reach the bottom at 20 seconds.
- Bend forward slightly and lift the dumbbell over one shoulder and place it on the floor, or have your spotter grasp the dumbbell from behind your neck and take it from you.

TIP

- Be alert in the bottom position of the negative-accentuated triceps extension, as the triceps is stretched across the elbow and the shoulder joints and thus vulnerable to strains. Move in and out of the bottom position very carefully, with no jerks.

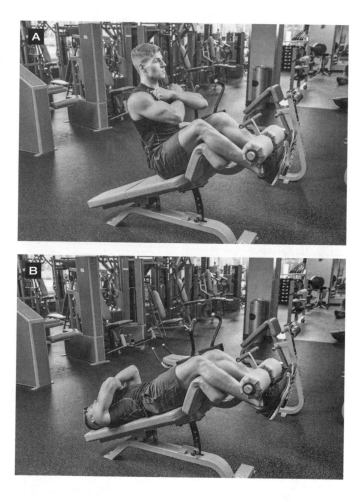

SIT-UP ON DECLINED BOARD

MUSCLES WORKED: Rectus abdominis, external obliques, and il-iopsoas (hip flexors)

PREPARATION

- Have a watch with a second hand—or, better yet, a big clock with a second hand—in plain sight, or have a spotter help with the counting.

- Place a long sit-up board in a stable position. Elevating the foot end will increase the difficulty of the negative-accentuated sit-up.
- Sit on the board and anchor your feet appropriately. Anchoring your feet brings into action more of your hip flexor muscles.
- Bend your knees and keep them bent through all phases.
- Start in the sitting-up position.
- Cross your arms over your chest and get ready to begin the first negative.

FIRST NEGATIVE
- Slowly lower your torso toward the backboard, inch by inch.
- Be halfway down at 10 seconds and three-quarters down at 15 seconds.
- Keep your midsection tight as you continue lowering.
- Reach the bottom at 20 seconds and get ready to begin the regular reps.

REGULAR REPS
- Contract your abdominals and hip flexors and move to the top position in 1 second and then return to the bottom in 2 seconds.
- Continue for 10 smooth reps.
- Hold the tenth rep at the top and get ready to begin the finish negative.

FINISH NEGATIVE
- Breathe freely as you start lowering your torso backward.
- Move slowly, inch by inch.
- Reach the bottom at 20 seconds.
- Ease off the board, stand, and relax.

TIPS
- This exercise requires good form. Practice keeping your face and neck relaxed throughout each phase. Do not reach with

your chin on the positive. Keep your knees bent at approximately 45 degrees throughout the exercise. Do not arch your back at the beginning, or end, on any phase.

- Make the negative-accentuated sit-up harder by elevating the foot end of the board, which raises your feet during the exercise. Also, you can increase the difficulty by removing your hands from your torso, cupping your fingers over your ears, and keeping your elbows in line with your head.

THE next two exercises, the Negative-Only Dip and the Negative-Only Chin-Up, are done in a way that involves only the negative phase of the movement. The idea, at the appropriate place in your routine, is to perform one negative repetition as slowly as possible. If you can do a 60-second lowering, which most trainees will have trouble doing, then you'll need to attach additional resistance to a belt around your waist.

While 60 seconds is indeed your goal, both of the negative-only exercises will be described using 30 seconds.

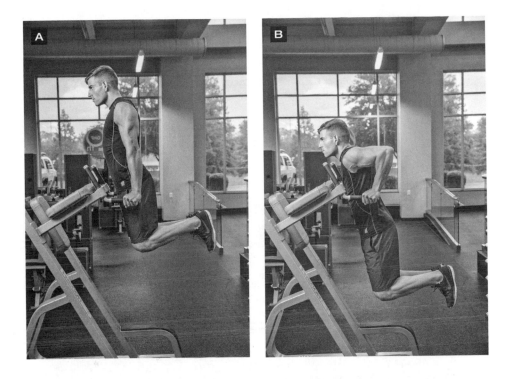

NEGATIVE-ONLY DIP

MUSCLES WORKED: Pectoralis major, deltoid, and triceps

PREPARATION

- Have a watch with a second hand—or, better yet, a big clock with a second hand—in plain sight, or have a spotter help with the counting.
- Place a sturdy chair or bench between the parallel bars, or use the built-in step or horizontal bar that some dipping bars provide.
- Climb to the top position and straighten your arms.
- Remove your feet from the chair and stabilize your body.

NEGATIVE ONLY

NOTE

The bottom of the finishing position occurs when the backs of your upper arms, when viewed from the side, dip below your elbows. Stop at this point.

- Lower your body by bending your arms slowly, ½ inch by ½ inch.
- Be halfway down at 15 seconds.
- Lean forward and keep your elbows tucked close to your body.
- Focus, breathe freely, and continue lowering yourself.
- Stop the movement at 30 seconds, or when the backs of your upper arms dip below your elbows.
- Place your feet back on the chair or attached bars.
- Exit the parallel bars and relax.

TIPS

- Be careful going into the bottom position. You want to feel the stretch more in your chest than in your shoulders. Do not go too low.
- Try to keep your face relaxed.

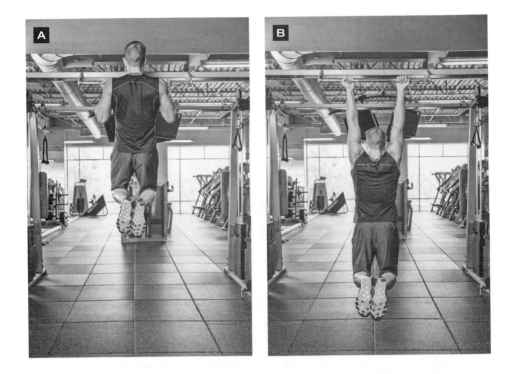

NEGATIVE-ONLY CHIN-UP

MUSCLES WORKED: Biceps, latissimus dorsi, and gripping muscles

PREPARATION

- Have a watch with a second hand—or, better yet, a big clock with a second hand—in plain sight, or have a spotter help with the counting.
- Place a sturdy chair or bench under an overhead chinning bar.
- Climb into the top position with your chin above the bar.
- Hold on to the bar with an underhand grip and your hands shoulder-width apart.
- Remove your feet from the chair or bench and stabilize your body.

NEGATIVE ONLY

- Lower your body by unbending your arms slowly, ½ inch by ½ inch.
- Be halfway down at 15 seconds.
- Lean back slightly and look up. Your knees should be bent and your ankles crossed.
- Continue to lower yourself until you reach a dead-hang position.
- Try to reach the bottom in 30 seconds.
- Place your feet back on the chair or bench and exit the chinning bar.

TIPS

- Prevent yourself from moving too fast by trying to stop and actually reverse the movement. You probably won't be able to reverse the movement, but just thinking about doing so will help you slow the descent.
- Grip the bar intensely at all times. You do not want your hands to slip.
- Try to keep your face, jaw, and neck relaxed. Doing so will help you concentrate more on the muscles you're trying to work.

MACHINE NEGATIVES

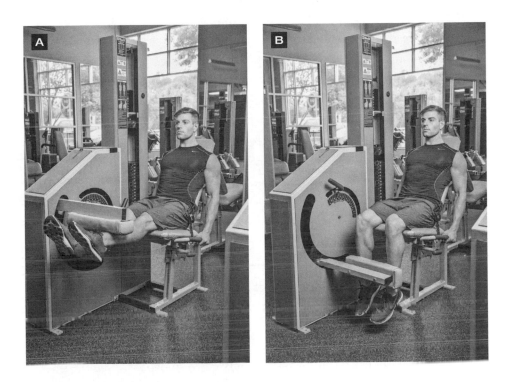

LEG EXTENSION

MUSCLES WORKED: Quadriceps

IMPORTANT NOTE: *Recently, there has been discussion that the leg extension is a dangerous exercise and as a result should not be used in most strength-training routines. Preliminary research has shown two problems: One, the leg extension tends to stress the anterior cruciate ligament within the knee, which can be problematic to anyone who has suffered ligament injuries to the knee. Two, the leg extension, with the movement arm perpendicular to the lower leg bones, tends to apply shear forces to the knee joint.*

As a consequence, some researchers and trainers believe that compression forces from the leg press and the squat are more beneficial to the knee than shear forces from the leg extension.

I've applied the leg extension with thousands of trainees. Plus, I've used it in the rehabilitation of many knee injuries, including anterior cruciate injuries and after surgery. My fifty years of training experience have shown me that almost any strength-training machine or strength-training free-weight exercise, if used incorrectly—which usually means fast and jerky with too much resistance—can cause, or lead to, an injury. On the other hand, almost any machine or exercise, if applied correctly—such as in the negative-accentuated style described in this book—can be a beneficial and productive way to increase muscle size and strength.

If you currently have a knee problem and want to play it safe, the leg extension machine may not be the best option for you, unless your healthcare professional recommends that you use it. The leg extension remains an important strength-building exercise that offers benefits to the quadriceps that other exercises cannot supply.

PREPARATION

- Have a watch with a second hand—or, better yet, a big clock with a second hand—in plain sight, or have a spotter help with the counting.
- Sit in the machine and place your feet and ankles behind the bottom roller pad.
- Align your knee joints with the axis of rotation of the movement arm.
- Fasten the seat belt, if one is provided, securely across your hips to keep your buttocks from rising.
- Lean back and stabilize your upper body by grasping the handles or the sides of the machine. With your spotter's assistance, efficiently lift the movement arm to the top position and pause.

FIRST NEGATIVE
- Begin lowering the movement arm slowly, inch by inch.
- Try to be halfway down at 10 seconds and three-quarters down at 15 seconds.
- Keep your focus.
- Be at the bottom at 20 seconds. Turn the movement around smoothly and get ready to begin the regular reps.

REGULAR REPS
- Straighten your legs smoothly in 1 second.
- Pause briefly and lower the resistance in 2 seconds.
- Continue for 10 repetitions.
- Lean back, not forward, as your legs straighten.
- Hold the ten rep at the top and stabilize your body for the finish negative.

FINISH NEGATIVE
- Lower the movement arm slowly, inch by inch.
- Be halfway down at 10 seconds and three-quarters down at 15 seconds.
- Relax your face and emphasize your breathing out.
- Fight for the last few seconds and set the weight down at 20 seconds.
- Be careful as you exit the machine.

TIPS
- Keep your feet relaxed during all phases of the leg extension. Do not extend or flex your toes. Keep them pointing straight ahead in a neutral position.
- Do not move your head forward or side to side.
- Practice smooth turnarounds at both ends of the exercise.

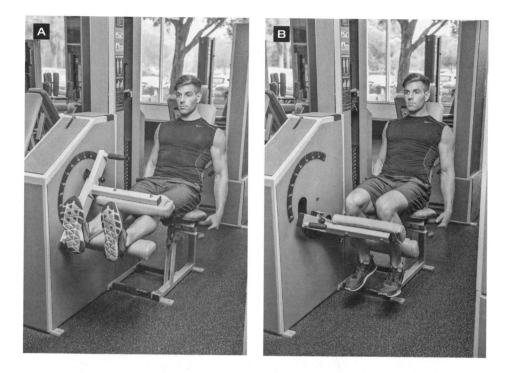

LEG CURL

MUSCLES WORKED: Hamstrings

NOTE:

There are several versions—prone, seated, and kneeling—of the leg curl machine. The one described here is performed in a seated position.

PREPARATION

- Have a watch with a second hand—or, better yet, a big clock with a second hand—in plain sight, or have a spotter help with the counting and initial lifting.
- Sit on the front part of the leg curl seat.
- Adjust the front part of the movement arm, slide your right and left feet into position, and make sure your knees are parallel to

the axis of rotation of the movement arm that is marked on the right machine panel.

- Secure the movement arm in place. The top pad should be on your shin and the bottom pad below your calf.
- Curl the movement arm efficiently to the contracted position, by yourself or with a spotter's assistance.
- Hold the contracted position briefly and get ready to begin the first negative.

FIRST NEGATIVE

- Lower the resistance slowly, inch by inch, by unbending your legs.
- Try to be halfway down at 10 seconds and three-quarters down at 15 seconds.
- Reach the resistance bottom at 20 seconds but do not rest. Turn the resistance around smoothly and get ready to begin the regular reps.

REGULAR REPS

- Curl the resistance arm smoothly in 1 second to the contracted position and lower it in 2 seconds to the bottom.
- Do 10 repetitions, in good form.
- Hold the tenth repetition in the contracted position and stabilize your body for the finish negative.

FINISH NEGATIVE

- Lower the resistance slowly, inch by inch.
- Be halfway down at 10 seconds.
- Keep your face relaxed and stay focused.
- Be three-quarters down at 15 seconds.
- Resist steadily and reach the bottom at 20 seconds.
- Readjust the movement arm by loosening it, slide your legs to the left, and exit the machine.

TIPS

- Keep your ankles dorsi-flexed, or with your toes pointed toward your knees, during both the negative and positive phases of the leg curl. This flexion of the ankle stretches your calves and allows for a greater range of motion of the hamstrings.
- Keep your face and neck relaxed during the movement.

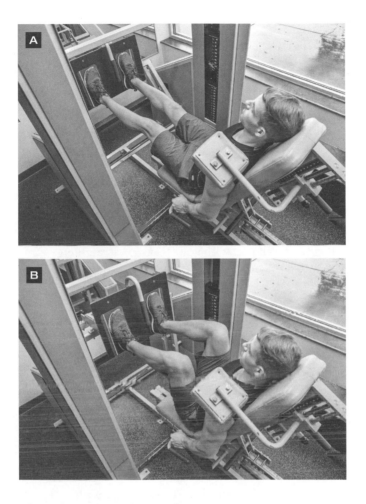

LEG PRESS

MUSCLES WORKED: Gluteals, quadriceps, and hamstrings

NOTE

There are many versions of the leg press machine. This one involves an adjustable seat carriage, seat back, and shoulder pads.

PREPARATION

- Have a watch with a second hand—or, better yet, a big clock with a second hand—in plain sight, or have a spotter help with the counting and initial lifting.
- Adjust the seat back and carriage to a comfortable setting until your knees—with your feet shoulder-width apart on the footboard—are near your chest. The closer the seat is to the footboard, the longer the range of motion and the harder the exercise.
- Note the seat carriage positions and adjust them to the same place each time you do the exercise.
- Grasp lightly the handles beside your hips.
- Press the footboard with your feet and straighten your hips and thighs. Get ready to begin the first negative.

FIRST NEGATIVE

- Lower the footboard slowly by bending your hips and knees.
- Try to be halfway down at 10 seconds and three-quarters down at 15 seconds.
- Turn the resistance around smoothly at 20 seconds. Do not stop and rest at the bottom. Barely touch and get ready to begin the regular reps.

REGULAR REPS

- Leg-press the footboard and weight smoothly to the top in 1 second and return it to the bottom in 2 seconds.
- Make sure the turnarounds at the bottom and top are carefully done. Do not bounce the weight at any time.
- Continue for 10 reps.
- Hold the tenth repetition at the top and get ready to begin the finish negative.

FINISH NEGATIVE

- Focus intensely and remember: You have more strength in the negative than the positive. You're still strong enough to do a final 20-second negative. Doing so successfully is the most important of these phases.

- Lower the footboard very slowly, inch by inch.
- Be halfway down at 10 seconds and three-quarters down at 15 seconds.
- Keep your face relaxed and breathe freely.
- The hardest portion is the last 5 seconds. Don't set the footboard on the stops until 20 seconds is completed.
- Readjust the seat carriage handle on the left side of the seat and move the seat backward until you can exit the machine easily.

TIPS

- The leg press is a very demanding exercise. Work diligently on keeping your movement slow and continuous.
- Practice keeping your face and neck relaxed.

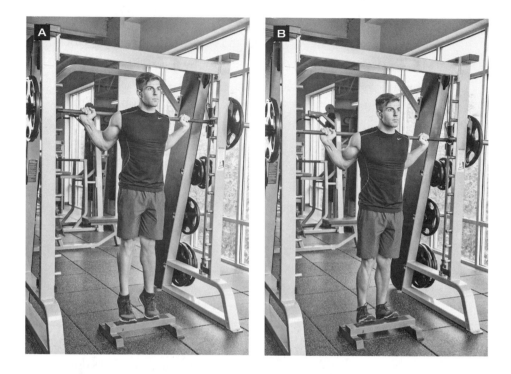

CALF RAISE

MUSCLES WORKED: Gastrocnemius and soleus

NOTE

There are various types of calf raise machines. The one described here is the standing version with a Smith machine that has a long barbell inside a fixed vertical plane of motion. The advantage of the Smith machine is that the long bar contains built-in hooks that engage into a series of slots or pegs that run the length of the vertical steel frame. Locate a sturdy block or a secure portable ledge to stand on. Wear rubber-soled shoes with treads on the bottom for better gripping with the soles of your feet.

PREPARATION

- Have a watch with a second hand—or, better yet, a big clock with a second hand—in plain sight, or have a spotter help with the counting and initial lifting.
- Place the block or portable ledge below the bar on the Smith machine. Adjust the level of the long bar to a couple of inches below your shoulder height.
- Step onto the block or ledge with the balls of your feet and place the bar on the back of your shoulders.
- Stand, rotate the bar forward, unrack it, and lift the resistance.
- Raise your heels, which contracts your calf muscles, and keep your knees stiff.
- Get as high as you can on your tiptoes and pause briefly before you begin the first negative.

FIRST NEGATIVE

- Lower your heels very slowly, ½ inch by ½ inch.
- Try to be halfway down at 10 seconds and three-quarters down at 15 seconds.
- Reach the bottom at 20 seconds, stretch briefly, and get ready to begin the regular reps.

REGULAR REPS

- Raise your heels in 1 second to the top and pause briefly.
- Do the negative phase in 2 seconds and pause briefly and stretch.
- Continue to perform the calf raise for 10 reps, in good form.
- Hold the tenth rep at the top and get ready to begin the finish negative.

FINISH NEGATIVE

- Lower your heels very slowly, ½ inch by ½ inch.
- Be halfway down at 10 seconds.

- Keep your knees locked. Do not bend them.
- Do a deep stretch at 20 seconds.
- Step down from the ledge gently, one foot at a time, rotate the handles backward, hook the bar in the slots, and relax.

TIPS

- Keep your knees straight during the movement, especially the bottom-stretch phases.
- If you do the repetitions smoothly and slowly, you'll get a deep burn in your posterior calf muscles—and probably some calf soreness over the next several days. Stretch your calves gently for relief.

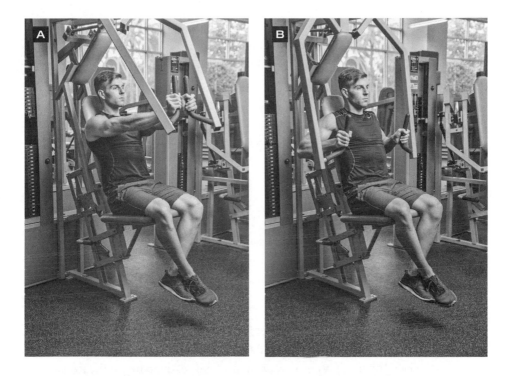

CHEST PRESS

MUSCLES WORKED: Pectoralis major, deltoid, and triceps

PREPARATION

- Have a watch with a second hand—or, better yet, a big clock with a second hand—in plain sight, or have a spotter help with the counting and initial lifting.
- Adjust the seat bottom on the machine so your hands can comfortably grasp the bottom handles of the movement arm.
- Note the numbers on the adjustment mechanisms. These numbers will allow you to duplicate the placements quickly during future workouts.
- Sit tall and grasp the handles. Keep your shoulder blades together throughout the movement.

- Straighten your elbows and move the weight stack efficiently to the top position by yourself or with assistance from your spotter. Get ready to begin the first negative.

FIRST NEGATIVE
- Lower the handles slowly, inch by inch.
- Be halfway down level at 10 seconds and three-quarters down at 15 seconds.
- Continue this deliberate lowering until 20 seconds have elapsed.
- Turn the resistance around smoothly and get ready to begin the regular reps.

REGULAR REPS
- Move out of the bottom smoothly and press the handles forward without jerking.
- Do the negative a little slower.
- Repeat the movement for 10 reps.
- Hold the tenth rep at extension and get ready to begin the finish negative.

FINISH NEGATIVE
- Lower the handles slowly, inch by inch.
- Stay in control and breathe freely. Keep your face relaxed.
- Be halfway down at 10 seconds.
- Be at the bottom at 20 seconds.
- Ease off the movement gradually. Remove your hands from the handles and relax.

TIPS
- Do not move your hips or arch your back excessively during the positive phase.
- Do not move your feet during either the negative or positive movements. Keep them grounded on the floor.

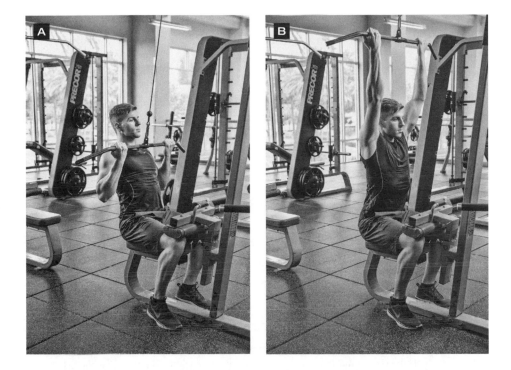

LAT MACHINE PULLDOWN

MUSCLES WORKED: Biceps and latissimus dorsi

PREPARATION

- Have a watch with a second hand—or, better yet, a big clock with a second hand—in plain sight, or have a spotter help with the counting.
- Sit and grasp the pulldown bar using an underhand grip with your hands shoulder-width apart.
- Stabilize your lower body properly.
- Pull the bar down to your chest efficiently and lift the resistance.
- Pause briefly, with the bar touching your upper chest. Your elbows should be down and back and holding steady. Get ready to begin the first negative.

FIRST NEGATIVE

- Unbend your arms and begin raising the bar slowly, inch by inch.
- Be halfway up at 10 seconds and three-quarters up at 15 seconds.
- Reach the top and stretch your arms at 20 seconds.
- Turn the resistance around smoothly and get ready to begin the regular reps.

REGULAR REPS

- Pull the bar down smoothly to your chest in 1 second.
- Raise the bar to the top in 2 seconds.
- Continue to lower and raise for 10 repetitions.
- Hold briefly at the bottom of the tenth repetition and get ready to begin the finish negative.

FINISH NEGATIVE

- Unbend your elbows and raise the bar slowly, inch by inch.
- Be halfway up at 10 seconds and three-quarters up at 15 seconds.
- Stay in control and breathe freely.
- Reach the top and stretch your arms and upper back at 20 seconds.
- Allow the resistance to bottom out on the weight stack, stand, and exit the machine.

TIP

- Keep your torso upright during the negative phases. Minimize body sway and practice strict form.

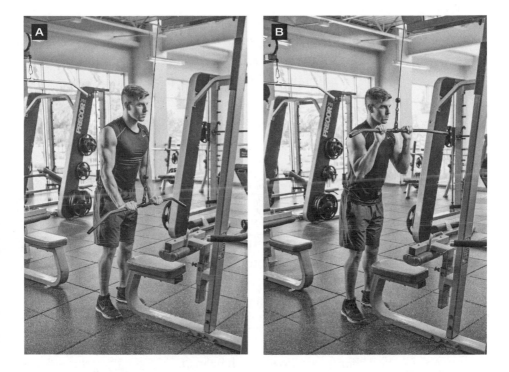

LAT MACHINE PUSHDOWN

MUSCLES WORKED: Triceps

PREPARATION

- Have a watch with a second hand—or, better yet, a big clock with a second hand—in plain sight, or have a spotter help with the counting.
- Stand up close to the machine.
- Grasp the handle using an overhand grip, with your hands ap proximately 6 inches apart.
- Push the bar down until your elbows are extended.
- Pause briefly and get ready to begin the first negative.

FIRST NEGATIVE

- Allow the bar to rise slowly, inch by inch.
- Be halfway up in 10 seconds and three-quarters up at 15 seconds.
- Be careful to not move your elbows. Keep them stationary at your sides.
- Reach the top at 20 seconds and get ready to begin the regular reps.

REGULAR REPS

- Push the bar and resistance to the fully extended position of your elbows in 1 second. Do not allow your elbows to move.
- Lower the resistance in 2 seconds.
- Repeat for 10 solid repetitions.
- Hold the tenth repetition at the bottom. Stabilize your body and get ready to begin the finish negative.

FINISH NEGATIVE

- Allow the bar to rise slowly, inch by inch.
- Be halfway up at 10 seconds.
- Reach the top at 20 seconds. You should feel a deep burn in your triceps.
- Allow the resistance to bottom out on the weight stack, stand, and exit the machine.

TIP

- This is a great exercise, but it's also easy to cheat. Do not allow your elbows to move once they are situated by your sides. Do not use momentum to initiate the regular reps. Keep your torso sway to a minimum. Force your triceps to maximum intensity.

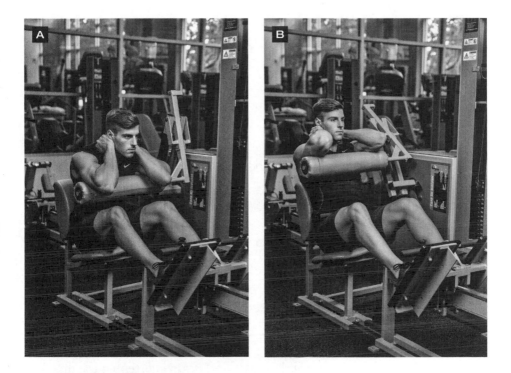

ABDOMINAL CRUNCH

MUSCLES WORKED: Rectus abdominis and external obliques

NOTE

Many different types of abdominal machines are manufactured today. I like the ones that are performed in an upright, seated position, with a pivot point at the midsection and a movement arm at the shoulders.

PREPARATION

- Have a watch with a second hand—or, better yet, a big clock with a second hand—in plain sight, or have a spotter help with the counting. Adjust the seat bottom so when you are seated your navel is parallel to the axis of rotation on the side.

- Fasten the seat belt, if there is one, across your hips, and place your feet on the platform.
- Place the movement arm roller pad securely under your arms.
- Get to the contracted position efficiently by leaning forward with your torso and elbows. Ready yourself for the first negative.

FIRST NEGATIVE
- Lean back, releasing your abdominal muscles slowly, ½ inch by ½ inch.
- Be halfway back at 10 seconds and three-quarters back at 15 seconds.
- Keep your face relaxed and breathe freely. Do not hold your breath.
- Reach the extended position and stretch at 20 seconds, and get ready to begin the regular reps.

REGULAR REPS
- Contract with your abdominals and begin shortening the distance between your lower ribs and pelvis.
- Keep the movement continuous by doing a 1-second positive followed by a 2-second negative.
- Be sure to breathe.
- Hold the contracted position of the tenth rep briefly and get ready to begin the finish negative.

FINISH NEGATIVE
- Release your abdominal muscles slowly, ½ inch by ½ inch, as you move backward.
- Keep your back rounded. Open your eyes and focus on the count.
- Be halfway back at 10 seconds and three-quarters back at 15 seconds. Arch your back slightly near the stretched position and allow the resistance to touch the weight stack at 20 seconds.
- Relax and exit the machine.

TIPS

- Keep your hips against the seat back throughout the movement by pushing with your thighs.
- Do not jut your chin forward at the start of the positive.
- Do not try to do a sit-up on this machine.
- Try to bring your rib cage closer to your pelvic girdle and reverse that action.
- Pull and release with the muscles in your midsection.

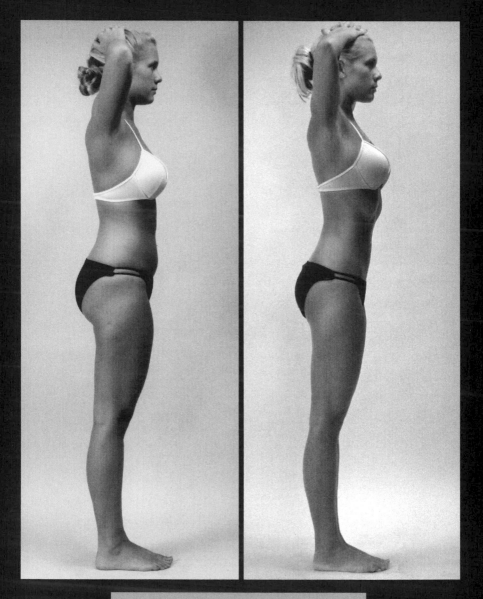

143 pounds   127 pounds

ASHLEY MEISNER, age 22, height 5'8"
AFTER 12 WEEKS
22.81 pounds of fat loss
6 inches off waist
6.81 pounds of muscle gain

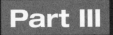

Part III

KILLING FAT SIX-WEEK PROGRAMS

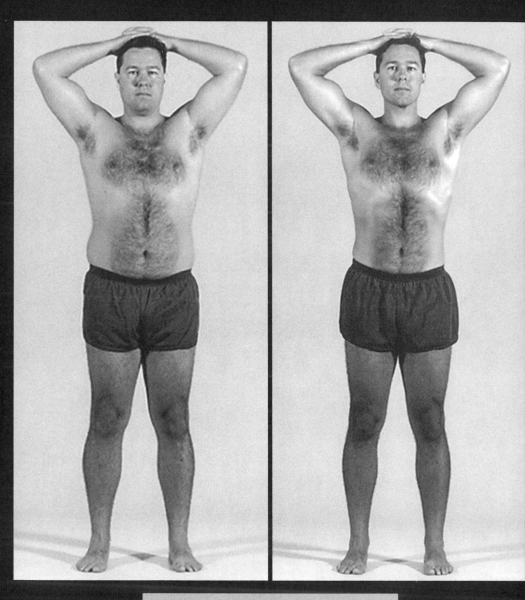

210.5 pounds   **175** pounds

JOE GENTRY, age 36, height 6'0"
AFTER 12 WEEKS
40.5 pounds of fat loss
6.75 inches off waist
5 pounds of muscle gain

10

BEFORE YOU BEGIN

IMPORTANT STEPS

Consult with Your Physician

BE SURE YOUR doctor knows you are going on the Killing Fat program. Let him examine this book so he understands what's involved. He may want to give you a physical if you have not had one in the last year.

There are a few people who should not try this program: children age fourteen and under; women who are pregnant or nursing; people with certain types of heart, liver, or kidney disease; diabetics; and those suffering from some types of arthritis. This should not be taken as an all-inclusive list. Some individuals should follow the course only with their physician's specific guidance and recommendations. Consult your doctor beforehand to play it safe.

Find a Friend to Go Through the Program with You

Although it is certainly possible to get great results going through the program by yourself, you'll probably lose more pounds and inches if you team up with a buddy—or several. You and your friend(s) should try to work out together, shop together, and share each other's problems.

The internet also offers a lot of opportunities for people near and far to go through this program together.

Take Your Measurements

You and your training partner can best take these measurements together. Wear a tight-fitting bathing suit (a two-piece bathing suit works best for women because it reveals the entire midsection).

	BEFORE	AFTER	DIFFERENCE
Body weight			
Right upper arm (hanging)			
Left upper arm (hanging)			
Chest (at nipple level)			
Belly, high (2 inches above navel, relaxed)			
Belly, middle (at navel level, relaxed)			
Belly, low (2 inches below navel, relaxed)			
Hips (at largest protrusion)			
Right thigh (just below butt crease)			
Left thigh (just below butt crease)			

Weigh yourself on your bathroom scale. Using a plastic tape measure, take all the other measurements standing, with your weight equally distributed on both feet. Apply the tape firmly, without compressing your skin, and keeping it parallel to the floor. Record the measurements to the nearest .125 inch. You'll be taking waist measurements at three levels: high (2 inches above your navel), middle (at your navel), and low (2 inches below your navel). Some individuals lose their fat at a greater or lesser degree from one or two of those levels, and you'll want to be aware of the difference.

Do the Pinch Test

For more than forty years, I've measured and determined body fat percentage and muscle gain using a Lange skinfold caliper, along with the formula and tables developed by Jackson and Pollock. It took me approximately a year to get skilled at the measurements and follow-up.

You, however, can get a fair estimate of your body fat percentage by doing the pinch test. For both men and women, this requires taking two measurements: the first on the back of the upper arm and the second beside the navel. Here's the procedure:

- Locate the first skinfold site on the back of the right upper arm (triceps area) midway between the shoulder and elbow. Let your arm hang loosely at your side.
- Grasp a vertical fold of skin between your thumb and forefinger. Pull the skin and fat away from the arm. Make sure the fold includes just skin and fat and no muscle.
- Measure with a ruler the thickness of the skin to the nearest .25 inch. Be sure to measure the distance between your thumb and forefinger. Sometimes the outer portion of the fold is thicker than the flesh grasped between the fingers. To avoid this, make sure the fold is level with the side of the thumb. Do not press the ruler against the skin. This will flatten it and make it appear thicker than it really is.
- Release the skin, record the triceps skinfold measurement on page 137, and repeat to take a second measurement at the same point.

- Calculate the average of the two triceps skinfold measurements and record this as well.
- Locate the second skinfold site, which is immediately adjacent to the right side of the navel.
- Grasp a vertical fold of skin between your thumb and forefinger and follow the same technique as for the triceps skinfold measurement.
- Release the skin, record the abdominal skinfold measurement, and repeat to take a second measurement at the same point.
- Calculate the average of the two abdominal skinfold measurements and record this.
- Add the averaged triceps skinfold measurement to the averaged abdominal skinfold measurement. This is your combined total.
- Estimate your body fat percentage from the chart on page 137 and record it above on the same page.
- Multiply your current body weight by your body fat percentage to determine how many pounds of fat you are carrying and record this as well.
- At the completion of the six-week program, take these measurements again to determine your current body fat percentage.

Determining Fat Loss and Muscle Gain

- Subtract your "after" weight from your "before" weight to find your total weight lost.
- Multiply your "before" body fat percentage by your "before" body weight; do the same for your "after" measurements. The difference between the two numbers is your total fat loss. For example, if a man weighed 208 pounds with 32 percent body fat at the start of the program, that's 66.56 pounds of fat. If he completed the program at 181 pounds at 18 percent body fat, that's 32.58 pounds of fat. The difference between 66.56 and 32.58 is 33.98 pounds.

- To determine your total muscle gain, subtract your fat loss from your total weight loss. In the example above, where fat loss equaled 33.98 pounds and weight loss was 27 pounds, 6.98 pounds of muscle were gained.

Fat comprises more than 25 percent of most Americans' body weight. An ideal amount of body fat is 12 percent for most men and 18 percent for most young women. Lean, athletic men and women may desire to lower their ideal figures by another 5 or 6 percentage points.

PINCH-TEST MEASUREMENTS

	BEFORE			AFTER			DIFFERENCE
	1ST	2ND	AVG	1ST	2ND	AVG	
Right triceps							
Right abdominal							
Combined Total							
Body fat percentage							
Fat pounds							
ESTIMATED PERCENTAGE OF BODY FAT							

SKINFOLD THICKNESS	BODY FAT PERCENTAGE	
TRICEPS + ABDOMINAL	MEN	WOMEN
.75 inch	5–9	8–13
1 inch	9–13	13–18
1.25 inches	13–18	18–23
1.5 inches	18–22	23–28
1.75 inches	22–27	28–33
2.25 inches	27–32	33–38
2.75 inches	32–37	38–43

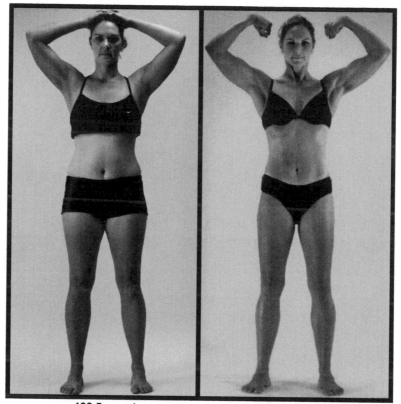

160.5 pounds   **143.5** pounds

JULIE MCGINLEY, age 38, height 5'7"
AFTER 12 WEEKS
22.34 pounds of fat loss
4.75 inches off waist
5.34 pounds of muscle gain

Take Full-Body Photographs

There is no better way to evaluate your current condition than to have full-body photographs taken of yourself in bicycle shorts or a tight bathing suit. Digital cameras and iPhones are easy to use. Here are the best procedures to follow:

- Wear solid-colored bicycle shorts or a tight-fitting bathing suit.
- Stand against an uncluttered, light-colored background.
- Direct the person with the camera to move away from you until they can see your entire body in the viewfinder. It's best that they be seated 15 to 20 feet from you, with the camera approximately 3 feet off the floor and turned for a vertical, or "portrait," format. They can zoom in as needed with the camera lens so your body fills the frame.
- Stand relaxed for two pictures: front, back, and right side. Do not try to suck in your stomach.
- Interlace your fingers and place them on top of your head so the contours of your torso are plainly visible. Keep your feet 8 inches apart for the front and back shots, but stand with them together for the side picture. (You can also take a double-arm biceps pose from the front and back.)
- Download the digital "Before" photos to your computer. Crop the best ones tightly to 3 by 6 inches.
- Take your "After" photos six weeks later, following the same directions, wearing the same bathing suit, and using the same camera.
- Download the images and crop them to the same size as your "Before" photos. Your height in both sets of photos should be the same.

Check Out Your Favorite Supermarket

The eating plan in chapter 11, "The No-Fuss Eating Option," is the simplest one I've ever designed. It also requires the least amount of preparation. Chapter 12, "The Cook-at-Home Eating Option," includes quick-and-easy recipes that you can make yourself using foods you can pick up from any supermarket.

Use Measuring Spoons, Cups, and a Kitchen Scale

Most people overestimate 3 ounces of deli-type ham, ½ cup of fat-free milk, or 2 tablespoons of sweet pickle relish. Such practices lead to inaccurate calorie counting and inefficient fat loss. It is important to become familiar with and correctly use measuring spoons, cups, and food scales.

Most of these items can be purchased inexpensively online or at local stores. With food scales, however, you'd be well-advised to spend more money to purchase a battery-operated digital scale instead of the less expensive spring-loaded analog type.

Take a Multivitamin with Minerals Each Day

While you're eating a reduced-calorie diet, you should take one multivitamin that includes minerals each morning. Study the label, however, and make sure no nutrient exceeds 100 percent of the RDA. High-potency supplements and super-stress formulas are a waste of money. It's also a good idea to consult your doctor before consuming any supplement.

Examine the Menus, Recipes, and Shopping Lists

Glance through the Killing Fat menus, recipes, and shopping lists in chapters 11 and 12 for an overview of what you'll be eating during the six-week program. Your results will be more effective if you plan ahead. One important concept to keep in mind is that your caloric intake will decrease slightly (by 100 calories) at the start of weeks 3 and 4, and again before weeks 5 and 6.

Get Serious, Trust the Process, Be Happy

You've done your tests, taken your measurements, made certain purchases, and familiarized yourself with what to expect. Now it's time to get serious. It's time to lose significant pounds and inches.

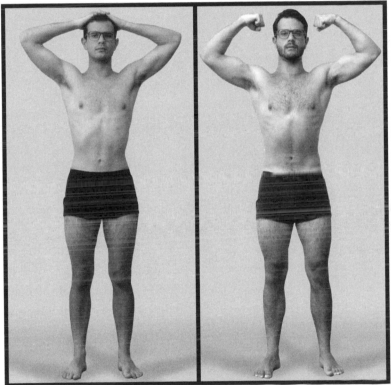

139.5 pounds   **155** pounds

BRANDEN MEDARY, age 21, height 5'8"
AFTER 12 WEEKS
(on muscle-building program only)
2.375 inches added on arms, **2.75** inches on chest
3.75 inches added on thighs
15.5 pounds of muscle gain

11

THE NO-FUSS EATING OPTION

KEEP IT SIMPLE

PUBLISHED *THE NAUTILUS DIET* in 1987. It contained a ten-week eating plan that provided seventy-two recipes. Each day, quite a bit of cooking was required.

Around the same time, Lean Cuisine frozen meals were created by Nestlé as a healthy alternative to some of their higher-calorie frozen selections. Because of the word *lean* in the title, the FDA required that they contain less than 10 grams of fat per serving. It didn't take long for other food manufacturers to jump into the lower-calorie, frozen-meal market. Also, by the mid-1990s, 50 percent of the households in the United States owned a microwave oven, which definitely facilitated the cooking process.

In 2014, I published *The Body Fat Breakthrough*, which had no recipes for the first six weeks. The primary cooking was frozen microwave meals that took 5 minutes at most to prepare. In fact, the test panelist who dropped the greatest number of fat pounds out of 145 subjects went through the program for thirty consecutive weeks and never cooked a single meal from a recipe. Instead, he chose from a comprehensive menu of more than one hundred frozen, microwavable, packaged meals.

In the last four years, however, there has been a resurgence of interest in cook-at-home meals made from recipes and less interest in packaged microwavable meals. To that end, chapter 12 covers the cook-at-home option and includes many tasty, low-calorie recipes for your enjoyment. I also include a specific fourteen-day meal plan in chapter 14 that will help you organize your low-calorie eating efficiently.

Frozen, Microwavable Meals

Numerous magazine articles and books would have you believe that processed foods are bad for you. Processing, they claim, sacrifices many nutrients, and the added chemicals may be dangerous. But remember, as I noted in chapter 5, that most foods, especially vegetables and fruits, are naturally packed with chemicals.

Recently, scientists at the University of Georgia and the University of California at Davis found in separate studies that frozen vegetables and fruits were just as nutritious as their fresh counterparts. In fact, the California research revealed that vitamin content was higher in some frozen foods, including broccoli, corn, green beans, and blueberries, because the freezing process keeps the nutrients of just-harvested food intact, while fresh produce may sit in transport or supermarkets for days, losing nutrients along the way.

I have no financial arrangement of any kind with Lean Cuisine or its parent company, Nestlé. Since the late 1980s, I've included Lean Cuisine meals (as well as meals made by Healthy Choice, Michelina's, and Weight Watchers) as choices in my diet programs. I've consistently found Lean Cuisine to be tasty, varied, nutritious, economical, and adaptable to my daily macronutrient breakdown of 50 percent carbohydrates, 25 percent proteins, and 25 percent fats.

Today, Lean Cuisine has more than one hundred frozen selections, classified under breakfasts, lunches, and dinners, which you can review on their website. The majority of these meals range between 250 and 400 calories. Also, they have broadened their scope to include meals that are vegetarian, gluten-free, and free of preservatives or artificial flavors. Most of the Lean Cuisine dinners contain less than 500 mg of sodium. (For context, the FDA recommends consuming no more than 2,300 milligrams of sodium per day.)

Automatic Success

I've found that diets that are complicated and require time-consuming food shopping and preparation are difficult for most people to maintain. That's why, for the first two weeks especially, I recommend that you avoid variety, repeat meals you really like, and use frozen microwavable meals for dinner to automate calorie and portion control.

I've made every attempt to use current, popular brand names and calorie counts, which are listed in the menus. But as you probably know, products are frequently changed, modified, and discontinued. If a listed food choice is not available in your area, you'll have to substitute something similar. Become a label reader at your supermarket. For the latest frozen, microwavable meals, and for possible dinner substitutions, visit:

- Leancuisine.com
- Michelinas.com
- Healthychoice.com

Each day, you will choose a limited selection of foods for breakfast and lunch. Ample variety during your evening meal, however, will make your daily eating interesting and enjoyable. Also, the eating plan includes snacks to keep your energy high and your hunger low.

You may have a noncaloric beverage with your main meals. Noncaloric beverages are any type of water—tap, bottled, carbonated, or flavored—with no calories.

Begin week 1 on Monday and continue through Sunday. Week 2 is a repeat of week 1. Calories for each food are noted in parentheses.

Shopping List

The quantities for one week of the listed foods will depend on your specific selections. Review your choices and adjust the shopping list accordingly. Remember to check nutrition information on products you buy so you can carefully follow the serving sizes in the menus. It may be helpful for you to photocopy this list each week before doing your shopping.

STAPLES

Mustard

Meal replacement shakes

Milk, fat-free

Almonds, whole, unsalted

Hellmann's Mayonnaise, light

Noncaloric beverages: water, diet soft drinks, tea, and coffee

GRAINS

Thomas' Hearty Grains whole wheat bagels

Thomas' English muffins

Whole wheat bread

Microwave popcorn, light

FRUITS

Apples (3-inch diameter)

Bananas (7 inches long)

Dried apricots

Prunes

Raisins

Cantaloupe (5-inch diameter)

VEGETABLES

Lettuce

Tomatoes

V8 juice

Corn, whole kernel, canned, no salt added

Sweet peas, canned

Three-bean salad, canned

Sweet pickle relish

DAIRY

cream cheese, low-fat

cheese, fat-free

flavored yogurt, light or fat-free

Breakstone's 100-Calorie Cottage Doubles

MEAT AND EGGS

White turkey meat, deli-style, thinly sliced

Ham, deli-style, thinly sliced

Large eggs

Tuna, canned, chunk light in water

FROZEN MICROWAVABLE DINNERS OR ENTRÉES

Black Bean with Red Quinoa Soup (Campbell's Well Yes!) (can)

Roasted Turkey Breast (Lean Cuisine Comfort)

Chicken Fettuccini (Lean Cuisine Favorites)

Santa Fe–Style Rice & Beans (Lean Cuisine Favorites)

Butternut Squash Ravioli (Lean Cuisine Marketplace)

Orange Chicken (Lean Cuisine Marketplace)

Tortilla Crusted Fish (Lean Cuisine Marketplace)

Creamy Rigatoni with Broccoli & Chicken (Michelina's Lean Gourmet)

Three Cheese Ziti (Michelina's Lean Gourmet)

Women consume 1,400 calories a day.

Men consume 1,600 calories a day.

BREAKFAST = 300 CALORIES

Choose one—bagel, muffin, or shake—
and a noncaloric beverage.

Bagel

1 whole wheat bagel (Thomas' Hearty Grains), toasted (240)

2 tablespoons light cream cheese (60)

English Muffin

1 English muffin (Thomas'), toasted (120)

1 hard-boiled egg (78)

4 dried apricots (70)

To drink: 1 (5.5-ounce) can V8 juice (30)

Shake

Blend until smooth:

2 scoops protein shake powder (Metabolic Drive) (220), or other
protein powder or shake mix or equivalent calories

1 medium banana (80)

1½ cups cold water

MIDMORNING SNACK = 100 CALORIES

Choose one:

1 cup light or fat-free flavored yogurt (100)

14 unsalted almonds (100)

1 apple (100)

2 cups light microwave popcorn (100)

LUNCH = 300 CALORIES

Choose one (sandwich or soup) and a noncaloric beverage.

HAM OR TURKEY SANDWICH (300)

2 slices whole wheat bread (140)

1 to 2 tablespoons classic mustard (0)

3 ounces thinly sliced deli-style ham or turkey (90)

1 ounce fat-free cheese (1½ slices) (50)

2 slices tomato (10)

2 lettuce leaves (10)

Soup: 1 (16.3-ounce) can Campbell's Well Yes! Black Bean with Red Quinoa Soup (280)

Men: Add 100 calories:

1 cup V8 juice (50)

7 unsalted almonds (50)

MIDAFTERNOON SNACK = 200 CALORIES

Choose two:

1 cup light or fat-free flavored yogurt (100)

1 (3.9-ounce) container Breakstone's Cottage Doubles, various flavors (100)

14 unsalted almonds (100)

1 apple (100)

2 cups light microwave popcorn (100)

DINNER = 300 CALORIES

Choose one entrée and a noncaloric beverage.

Santa Fe–Style Rice & Beans (Lean Cuisine Favorites) (290)

Orange Chicken (Lean Cuisine Marketplace) (310)

Tortilla Crusted Fish (Lean Cuisine Marketplace) (300)

Three Cheese Ziti (Michelina's Lean Gourmet) (280)

Men: Add 100 calories:

1½ slices whole wheat bread (105)

EVENING SNACK = 200 CALORIES

Choose two:

1 cup light or fat-free flavored yogurt (100)

1 (3.9-ounce) container Breakstone's Cottage Doubles, various flavors (100)

14 unsalted almonds (100)

1 apple (100)

2 cups light microwave popcorn (100)

Killing Fat Eating Plan for Weeks 3 and 4 and Weeks 5 and 6

WOMEN: **Weeks 3 and 4** = 1,300 calories a day
Eliminate one Midafternoon Snack (–100 calories) from Week 1 and 2 menus.

Weeks 5 and 6 = 1,200 calories a day
Eliminate one Evening Snack (–100 calories) from Week 3 and 4 menus.

MEN: **Weeks 3 and 4** = 1,500 calories a day
Eliminate one Midafternoon Snack (–100 calories) from Week 1 and 2 menus.

Weeks 5 and 6 = 1,400 calories a day
Eliminate one Evening Snack (–100 calories) from Week 3 and 4 menus.

Substitutions
One of the following may be substituted for a 300-calorie lunch:

CHEF SALAD

In a large bowl, mix:

2 cups chopped lettuce (20)
2 ounces chopped cooked chicken or turkey, white meat only (80)
2 ounces fat-free cheese, grated (100)
4 slices tomato, chopped (28)
1 tablespoon fat-free dressing (8)
1 slice whole wheat bread, toasted (70)

SANDWICH FROM SUBWAY

6-inch turkey breast & Black Forest ham on 9-grain wheat bread with plenty of raw vegetables and no oil-based dressings (300)

One of the following may be substituted for a 100-calorie snack:

FRUITS

5 prunes (100)

1 ounce raisins (82)

½ cantaloupe (5-inch diameter) (94)

ENERGY BARS

Most of the popular energy bars—such as ZonePerfect, PowerBar, Odwalla, and Clif—may be used as snacks. Their calories, however, range from 210 to 240; so slightly less than ½ bar may be applied as one selection.

One of the following may be substituted for a 300-calorie dinner:

TUNA SALAD WITH CORN AND PEAS (260)

In a large bowl, mix:

½ (5-ounce) can chunk light tuna in water, drained (50)

½ cup canned no-salt-added whole kernel corn (4 ounces) (60)

½ cup canned sweet peas (4 ounces) (60)

2 tablespoons sweet pickle relish (40)

1 tablespoon Hellmann's light mayonnaise (50)

1 tablespoon Dijon mustard (0)

TUNA-BEAN DELIGHT (280)

In a large bowl, mix:

½ (5-ounce) can chunk light tuna in water, drained (50)

½ cup canned sweet peas (4 ounces) (60)

½ cup canned three-bean salad (4 ounces), drained (70)

½ apple, cored and chopped (50)

1 tablespoon Hellmann's light mayonnaise (50)

ROASTED TURKEY BREAST (Lean Cuisine Comfort) (260)

CHICKEN FETTUCCINI (Lean Cuisine Favorites) (290)

BUTTERNUT SQUASH RAVIOLI
(Lean Cuisine Marketplace) (260)

CREAMY RIGATONI WITH BROCCOLI & CHICKEN
(Michelina's Lean Gourmet) (270)

12

THE COOK-AT-HOME EATING OPTION

KILLING FAT RECIPES

A **LOT OF PEOPLE** are into "eating clean." They try to avoid processed and packaged foods and eat organic beef, free-range chicken, whole-grain breads, and fresh vegetables and fruits. Sure, I like an organic, fresh, crisp apple and a warm slice of homemade whole wheat bread with Irish grass-fed butter. But I'm also a realist when it comes to food and nutrition. Not everyone has access to a farm stand or the income to buy organic foods every week. And cooking meals from fresh, whole ingredients every day is not something many of us can fit into our busy lives.

For simplicity's sake, I advocate frozen meals and packaged foods (see chapter 11 for more on this). They provide almost instant portion and caloric control, making it easy to stick to the daily meal plans in the previous chapter.

But I wanted to offer some alternatives for those who would like to make their own meals. Here you'll find twenty-two recipes, many of which were contributed by Gainesville Health & Fitness test panelists. Each listing is delicious and filling, and falls within the calorie guidelines.

Billie DeNunzio, an old friend who went through my first Nautilus

Diet program in 1985 and lost 25 pounds of fat, is an award-winning chef and the director of Eastside High School's Culinary Arts Academy in Gainesville. Chef DeNunzio worked through all the recipes in this chapter, including the recipes provided by test panelists, and formulated each one according to the nutritional requirements of the Killing Fat eating plan.

If you'd like to follow a specific seven- or fourteen-day meal plan incorporating these recipes, check out chapter 14. Another way to include these dishes is to follow the chapter 11 guidelines for breakfast, lunch, and snacks, but cook one of these recipes for dinner. A week or two later, you can add breakfasts and lunches from recipes in this chapter. Some dieters who enjoy cooking still like to have the frozen meals handy for emergencies. They work well if you are in a hurry and running late.

BLACK BEAN VEGGIE PATTIES

Preheat the oven to 375°F or heat a grill to medium-high.

In a large bowl, mash the black beans with a fork until thick and pasty.

Put the bell pepper, onion, and garlic in a colander set in the sink and squeeze to remove as much liquid as possible. Add the onion mixture to the mashed black beans and stir to combine.

In a medium bowl, stir together the eggs, chili powder, cumin, salt, black pepper, and Thai chili sauce.

Add the egg mixture to the bean mixture and stir to combine.

Mix in the bread crumbs until the mixture is sticky and holds together.

Divide the mixture into four patties.

If baking, place the patties on a baking sheet and bake for about 10 minutes on each side. If grilling, place the patties on foil and grill about 8 minutes on each side.

Place the patties on a whole wheat bun (190 calories) and add toppings like mustard, tomatoes, pickles, onions, and lettuce (40 calories) . . . and you have a tasty 300-calorie burger.

1 16-ounce can black beans, drained, rinsed, and patted dry

½ green bell pepper, finely chopped

½ onion, finely chopped

3 garlic cloves, finely chopped

2 large eggs

1 tablespoon chili powder

1 teaspoon ground cumin

½ teaspoon kosher salt

¼ teaspoon freshly ground black pepper

1 teaspoon Thai chili sauce or sriracha

1 cup panko bread crumbs

4 whole wheat buns, for serving

Optional toppings: mustard, tomatoes, pickles, onions, lettuce

CALORIES PER SERVING 70
YIELD 4 servings
SERVING SIZE 10 ounces
PREPARATION TIME 20 minutes
TOTAL TIME 30 minutes

ROBUST TURKEY MEATBALL SOUP

8 ounces ditalini or other small pasta

½ cup canned diced tomato

32 ounces low-sodium chicken broth

1 cup small-diced carrots

1 cup chopped celery

32 fully-cooked frozen turkey meatballs

6 ounces Saffron Road Crunchy Chickpeas, for garnish

2 tablespoons grated Parmesan cheese, for garnish

CALORIES PER SERVING 246

YIELD 4 servings

SERVING SIZE 1¼ cups

PREPARATION TIME 20 minutes

TOTAL TIME 20 minutes

Bring a large pot of water to a boil. Add the pasta and cook according to the package directions until al dente, about 5 minutes. Remove from the heat and drain. Return the pasta to the pot and add the tomato.

In a medium sauce pot, heat the chicken broth over medium-high heat. Add the carrots and celery and cook for about 5 minutes, or until soft.

Add the frozen turkey meatballs and cook for 3 to 5 minutes, until warmed through.

Place 8 meatballs in the bottom of each of four soup bowls.

Add ¼ cup of the cooked pasta to each bowl.

Top with the hot consommé and veggies, ladling them gently into each bowl.

Garnish each serving with the crunchy chickpeas and cheese.

Serve immediately.

QUINOA PILAF WITH PISTACHIOS

In a fine-mesh sieve, rinse quinoa under cold water for about 1 minute and drain well.

In a medium saucepan, heat the olive oil over medium heat. Add the scallion whites, garlic, and bell pepper and cook, stirring, until tender, about 5 minutes.

Reduce the heat from medium to low, stir in the quinoa, and toast, stirring continuously, for 2 minutes.

Add the broth, cardamom, and 1½ cups water and bring to a boil.

Reduce the heat to low, cover, and simmer for 20 minutes, or until the liquid has been absorbed.

Remove from the heat; let stand for 5 minutes.

Fluff with a fork. Stir in the pistachios.

Garnish with the scallion greens and serve.

1 cup quinoa

2 tablespoons extra-virgin olive oil

4 scallions, chopped, white and green parts kept separate

3 garlic cloves, minced

½ cup red bell pepper, diced

1 cup reduced-sodium vegetable broth

¼ teaspoon ground cardamom

½ cup pistachios, chopped

CALORIES PER SERVING 143
YIELD 6 servings
SERVING SIZE 6 ounces
PREPARATION TIME 30 minutes
TOTAL TIME 30 minutes

CLASSIC DERBY COBB SALAD WITH TURKEY CUTLETS

DRESSING

- 2 tablespoons cider vinegar
- 1 teaspoon Dijon mustard
- 1 tablespoon extra-virgin olive oil
- 2 tablespoons water
- Kosher salt and pepper

SALAD

- 2 large eggs
- 1 pound turkey breast cutlets
- 1 teaspoon extra-virgin olive oil
- Kosher salt
- 8 cups baby spinach leaves (see Note)
- 4 slices reduced-sodium turkey bacon, cooked and crumbled
- ½ avocado, pitted, peeled, and diced
- 12 cherry tomatoes, halved
- 2 ounces blue cheese, crumbled
- 2 scallions, chopped

CALORIES PER SERVING 360
YIELD 4 servings
SERVING SIZE 10 ounces
PREPARATION TIME 10 minutes
TOTAL TIME 15 minutes

Make the dressing: In a small bowl, whisk together the vinegar, mustard, olive oil, and 2 tablespoons water until smooth. Season with salt and pepper and set aside.

Make the salad: Place the eggs in a medium saucepan and add cold water to cover by 1 inch. Bring the water to a boil over medium heat. Cover, remove from the heat, and let the eggs stand in the hot water for 10 minutes. Drain the eggs in a colander and cool under cold running water. Once cool, peel and chop the eggs; set aside.

Heat a skillet over medium-high heat for 2 minutes. Brush the turkey with the olive oil and sprinkle lightly with salt. Reduce the heat to medium-low, place the cutlets in the pan, and cook for 3 minutes on each side, then cook for about 3 minutes more, until the center of each cutlet is opaque and the juices run clear, or the internal temperature is 165°F. Remove the turkey from the pan and let cool, then cut into chunks.

In a large bowl, toss the spinach with 2 tablespoons of the dressing (whisk it again before using, if necessary), then divide the spinach among four individual plates.

On each plate, arrange one-quarter of the hard-boiled eggs, turkey, bacon, avocado, tomatoes, blue cheese, and scallions in a row on top of the lettuce. Drizzle the remaining dressing over the salads and season with salt and pepper.

NOTE: Chopped salad greens (iceberg lettuce, watercress, endives, and romaine lettuce) can be substituted for the baby spinach.

SWEET & SOUR THAI BEEF SALAD

10 ounces boneless beef strip or flank steak, 1½ inches thick (see Notes)

1 tablespoon corn oil, peanut oil, or other vegetable oil

Kosher salt and freshly ground black pepper

2 tablespoons fresh lime juice

2 tablespoons fish sauce

1 garlic clove, minced

1 teaspoon Thai or red serrano chile or jalapeño, seeded and minced (see Notes)

1 tablespoon brown sugar

1 cup radishes, thinly sliced

1 small red onion, thinly sliced, rinsed, and drained

1 medium kirby cucumber, thinly sliced

2 medium tomatoes, cored and cut into small wedges

¼ cup fresh mint leaves, coarsely chopped

10 fresh basil leaves, cut into chiffonade (see Notes)

4 cups thinly sliced romaine hearts (about 2 hearts)

CALORIES PER SERVING 192
YIELD 4 servings
SERVING SIZE 10 ounces
PREPARATION TIME 10 minutes
TOTAL TIME 15 minutes

Heat a grill to high or preheat the broiler.

Rub both sides of the steak with the oil and season with salt and pepper. Set aside.

In a large bowl, whisk together the lime juice, fish sauce, garlic, chile, and brown sugar; set aside 1 tablespoon for serving. (This sauce can be refrigerated, covered, for up to 2 weeks.)

In a separate large bowl, combine the radishes, onion, cucumber, tomatoes, mint, basil, and lettuce. Add the vegetables to the bowl with the dressing and toss well to combine.

Arrange the salad on a large platter.

Grill or broil the beef for 2 minutes, until rare to medium (it will continue to cook as it rests). (Steak is best rare to medium and still pink in the center.)

Transfer the steak to a cutting board and slice it as thinly as possible across the grain. Put the sliced steak in a bowl and toss with the reserved 1 tablespoon dressing.

Arrange the warm steak on top of the salad and serve.

NOTES: Roast beef from the deli counter can also be used; this saves time and effort but is more expensive.

If chile peppers are not available, you can substitute red pepper flakes.

To chiffonade the basil (or other fresh herbs or greens), stack the leaves, roll them up tightly like a cigar, then thinly slice the roll crosswise. This results in long, thin ribbons.

ZESTY LIME SHRIMP SALAD

2 teaspoons lime zest

1½ tablespoons fresh lime juice

2 tablespoons fresh cilantro, chopped, plus whole sprigs for garnish

1 scallion, finely chopped

1½ teaspoons hoisin sauce

½ teaspoon extra-virgin olive oil

¼ teaspoon minced garlic

Pinch of ground white pepper

8 ounces large shrimp, peeled and deveined (see Notes)

¼ cup diced red bell pepper

¼ cup chopped red onion

Bibb lettuce leaves, for serving

Lime slices, for garnish

CALORIES PER SERVING   150

YIELD   2 servings

SERVING SIZE   ½ cup

PREPARATION TIME   10 minutes

TOTAL TIME   40 minutes

In a large bowl, whisk together lime zest, lime juice, chopped cilantro, scallion, hoisin sauce, olive oil, garlic, and white pepper. Reserve 1 tablespoon of the mixture and set the rest aside. Set aside.

In a large nonstick skillet, heat 1 tablespoon of the reserved mixture over medium heat. Add the shrimp. Cook, tossing, for 2 to 3 minutes, until the shrimp are opaque.

Pour the lime mixture into a large zip-top freezer bag. Add the shrimp and bell pepper, seal, and turn to coat. Chill, turning occasionally, for 30 minutes.

Line each serving plate with lettuce leaves. Divide the shrimp among the plates, placing it on top of the lettuce. Spoon the marinade from the bag over the mixture.

Garnish with lime slices and fresh cilantro sprigs.

NOTES: Fresh fruit, such as avocado or mandarin oranges, would enhance this dish. Be sure to add approximately 50 calories to your total.

Add 1 teaspoon red pepper flakes for a little more heat.

To make this recipe even easier, purchase cooked and peeled shrimp. If using ready cooked shrimp, allow the mixture to marinate longer to enhance the flavor. If using frozen shrimp, allow the shrimp to thaw and rinse before combining it with the marinade.

SHIRATAKI SHRIMP SCAMPI FETTUCCINE

1 (8-ounce) package shirataki fettuccine

2 tablespoons extra-virgin olive oil

1 pound medium shrimp, peeled and deveined

4 garlic cloves, minced

½ teaspoon red pepper flakes

1 pint cherry tomatoes, halved

½ cup dry white wine

Juice of 1 lemon (2 to 3 tablespoons)

4 cups baby spinach

1 tablespoon unsalted butter

½ cup chopped fresh parsley

1 tablespoon lemon zest

Kosher salt and pepper

½ cup grated Parmesan cheese

CALORIES PER SERVING 336

YIELD 4 servings

SERVING SIZE 1 cup

PREPARATION TIME 10 minutes

TOTAL TIME 20 minutes

Bring a large pot of water to a boil.

Drain the noodles in a large sieve and rinse well under cold running water. Add them to the pot with the boiling water and cook for 2 to 3 minutes. (This step is important for removing the noodles' initial unpleasant odor.)

Drain the noodles.

Heat a large dry skillet over medium-high heat. Add the noodles and cook, turning them with tongs, for about 10 minutes. There will be a lot of steam—remove as much water as possible without drying them out. (This step is important for their texture.)

Transfer the noodles to a bowl.

In the same skillet, heat the olive oil over medium heat.

Add the shrimp and cook, stirring, until just cooked through and starting to turn pink. Transfer the shrimp to a large bowl and set aside.

Add garlic, red pepper flakes, tomatoes, wine, and lemon juice to skillet and cook over high heat for 2 minutes, or until the tomatoes start to soften.

Add the spinach and cook, stirring, for 1 minute, or until the spinach wilts.

Add the butter and cook, stirring, until melted, then return the shrimp and shirataki noodles to the pan and add the parsley and lemon zest. Taste and adjust the seasonings with salt and pepper. Remove from the heat immediately.

Transfer to a serving platter and serve immediately.

Sprinkle each serving with 2 tablespoons of the cheese.

NOTE: Shirataki noodles originated in Japan. They are thin, translucent, gelatinous noodles made from konjac root, also called white yam. Largely composed of water and glucomannan, a water-soluble dietary fiber, they are very low in digestible carbohydrates and calories, and high in fiber. They have little flavor of their own, but soak up the flavor of the dish, making them a great vehicle for sauces and toppings.

1　Gardein Chick'n Scallopini or other frozen vegan protein patty

½　cup canned black beans, drained

2　tablespoons prepared salsa

Kosher salt and pepper

1　cup arugula

1　slice Nature's Own Honey Wheat bread, toasted

CALORIES PER SERVING　310

YIELD　1 serving

PREPARATION TIME　10 minutes

TOTAL TIME　10 minutes

Lightly coat a nonstick skillet with cooking spray and heat over medium heat.

Add the veggie patty and cook until browned, 2 minutes on each side.

Add the black beans, then top with the salsa.

Cover and cook until the beans and salsa are warm, 1 to 2 minutes.

Season with salt and pepper.

Serve on a bed of arugula with the toast alongside.

GRILLED LEMON & ROSEMARY SHRIMP

What a great combination of flavors! Grilling the shrimp is a healthy way of cooking and keeps your kitchen clean while topping off the flavor. (The shrimp can also be broiled.)

Soak four 12-inch bamboo or wooden skewers in water for about 1 hour before using.

In a small bowl, whisk together the lemon juice, olive oil, basil, thyme, finely chopped rosemary, and garlic.

Add the shrimp and toss to coat with the marinade. Cover and refrigerate for 1 hour.

Heat a grill to medium-high or preheat the broiler. Drain the skewers.

Thread the shrimp onto the skewers, alternating with the lemon slices.

Season the skewers with salt and pepper. (At this point, the skewers can be refrigerated for 2 to 3 hours before cooking.)

Place the skewers on the grill over direct heat. Or, set the skewers on a baking sheet and place under the broiler. Grill or broil until the shrimp are opaque or light pink throughout, 2 to 3 minutes per side.

Garnish the shrimp with rosemary sprigs and serve with lemon wedges.

2 tablespoons fresh lemon juice

2 tablespoons extra-virgin olive oil

1 teaspoon dried basil

½ teaspoon dried thyme

2 tablespoons chopped fresh rosemary

2 garlic cloves, minced

1 pound extra-large shrimp (about 20), peeled and deveined

2 lemons, sliced ½ inch thick

Kosher salt and pepper

CALORIES PER SERVING 110

YIELD 4 servings

SERVING SIZE 1 skewer (5 shrimp)

PREPARATION TIME 10 minutes

TOTAL TIME 1 hour 15 minutes

SPAGHETTI SQUASH TURKEY BOLOGNESE

1 medium spaghetti squash, halved lengthwise and seeded

2 teaspoons extra-virgin olive oil

Kosher salt and pepper

2 ounces pancetta or bacon, chopped

½ cup chopped yellow onion

2 garlic cloves, minced

1 celery stalk, chopped

1 carrot, diced

1 pound 93% lean ground turkey

½ cup white wine

1½ teaspoons tomato paste

½ cup 1% milk

1 (28-ounce) can crushed tomatoes

¼ teaspoon red pepper flakes

½ teaspoon dried basil

½ teaspoon kosher salt

¼ teaspoon pepper

4 tablespoons grated Parmesan cheese

CALORIES PER SERVING   301

YIELD   4 servings

SERVING SIZE   10 ounces

PREPARATION TIME   25 minutes

TOTAL TIME   45 minutes

Preheat the oven to 400°F. Spray a baking sheet with cooking spray.

Brush the cut sides of the squash halves with olive oil and season generously with salt and black pepper. Place them cut-side down on the prepared baking sheet and roast until fork-tender, about 30 minutes. Remove from the oven and set aside to cool.

Meanwhile, in a large skillet, cook the pancetta over medium heat until the fat melts, about 3 minutes. Use a slotted spoon to transfer the pancetta to a plate and set aside.

Reduce the heat to medium-low and add the onion, garlic, celery, and carrot. Cook until soft, 5 to 6 minutes. Transfer to a bowl and set aside.

Raise the heat to medium-high and add the ground turkey. Cook, breaking up the meat with a wooden spoon, until no longer pink, 5 minutes.

Add the wine and cook until reduced by half, 2 to 3 minutes. Add the tomato paste, milk, crushed tomatoes, red pepper flakes, basil, and the onion mixture.

Bring to a simmer, reduce the heat to low, and cook until the turkey is cooked through and the sauce is thickened, 5 minutes. Season with salt and black pepper.

When the squash has cooled, use a fork to scrape the flesh from the skins in long, spaghetti-like strands.

For each serving, top 1 cup of the spaghetti squash "noodles" with ¾ cup of the sauce and sprinkle with 1 tablespoon of the cheese.

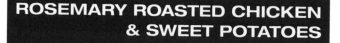

4 small bone-in, skin-on chicken breasts

1 tablespoon extra-virgin olive oil

3 sprigs fresh rosemary, chopped, or 1 tablespoon dried

½ teaspoon kosher salt

½ teaspoon pepper

4 sweet potatoes, cut into 2- to 3-inch cubes

1 large red onion, sliced ½ inch thick

CALORIES PER SERVING 332

YIELD 4 servings

SERVING SIZE 10 ounces

PREPARATION TIME 10 minutes

TOTAL TIME 40 minutes

Preheat the oven to 400°F.

Place the chicken breasts in a large bowl and drizzle with the olive oil. Sprinkle with the rosemary. Season with salt and pepper.

Use your fingers to loosen the skin over the breasts and spread a little of the seasoning under the skin. Place the chicken breasts skin-side-down in a 9- by 13-inch baking pan.

Arrange the sweet potatoes and sliced onion around the chicken breasts.

Roast, uncovered, for 30 minutes, until the chicken is no longer pink in the center and the juices run clear; an instant-read thermometer inserted into the center of a chicken breast should read 165°F. Remove from the oven.

Serve each breast with one-quarter of the sweet potatoes and onion, with the juices from the pan spooned over the top.

SKIRT STEAK SALAD

In a medium skillet, heat 1 tablespoon of the olive oil over medium-high heat.

Add the walnuts, onion, and shallot and cook about 1 minute. Transfer the walnut mixture to a plate and set aside.

Season the steak with the salt, pepper, and garlic powder. Add the steak to the hot pan and sear until browned on the bottom, about 5 minutes, then turn and sear until browned on the second side, 3 to 5 minutes more. Transfer the steak to a cutting board and let rest for 5 minutes.

In a large bowl, combine the arugula, walnut mixture, and remaining 2 tablespoons olive oil and toss to coat. Divide the arugula mixture between two plates.

Thinly slice the steak across the grain and divide it between the plates.

Top with the cherry tomatoes and feta.

3 tablespoons extra-virgin olive oil

¼ cup walnuts, chopped

½ red onion, thinly sliced

1 shallot, thinly sliced

¾ pound skirt steak

½ teaspoon kosher salt

¼ teaspoon pepper

¼ teaspoon garlic powder

6 cups baby arugula

1 cup cherry tomatoes, halved

¼ cup crumbled feta cheese

CALORIES PER SERVING 425 (men); 284 calories (women)
YIELD 2 servings
SERVING SIZE 3 cups for men; 2 cups for women
PREPARATION TIME 10 minutes
TOTAL TIME 25 minutes

EGG WHITE OMELET

4 egg whites (about 4 ounces)

Kosher salt and pepper

OPTIONAL INGREDIENTS

1 tablespoon sautéed diced onion

1 tablespoon sautéed diced bell pepper

1 tablespoon sautéed diced mushroom

2 ounces chopped frozen spinach, thawed and squeezed dry

Whole wheat toast, for serving

CALORIES PER SERVING 109

YIELD **1 serving**

PREPARATION TIME **5 minutes**

TOTAL TIME **10 minutes**

In a medium bowl, whisk the egg whites and a pinch of salt and pepper until frothy.

Lightly coat a medium nonstick skillet or omelet pan with cooking spray and heat the skillet over medium heat.

Add the egg whites, swirling to evenly cover the bottom of the pan. Cook for 2 minutes, allowing the egg to set.

Use a rubber spatula to lift the eggs up and let the runny uncooked egg flow underneath.

Spoon whatever filling you want onto half the omelet, cover the pan for about 1 minute, then fold the unfilled half of the omelet over the fillings and slide it onto a serving plate, over toast, if desired.

HOMEMADE GRANOLA

Preheat the oven to 300°F. Spray a rimmed baking sheet with cooking spray or line it with parchment paper.

In a large bowl, stir together the oats, almonds, wheat germ, sunflower seeds, coconut, cinnamon, nutmeg, and salt. Set aside.

In a small saucepan, whisk together the oil, maple syrup, honey, and vanilla. Bring to a boil, then immediately remove from the heat and pour over the oat mixture.

Mix and stir with a wooden spoon until all the oats and nuts are coated.

Spread the mixture evenly over the prepared baking sheet.

Bake until crispy, golden brown, and toasted, about 20 minutes, stirring once halfway through.

Remove from the oven. *Once cool, add the dried fruit of your choice.*

Store the granola in an airtight container in a cool, dry place for up to 2 weeks.

4 cups old-fashioned oats (not instant/quick-cooking)

1 cup sliced almonds

¾ cup wheat germ

½ cup hulled sunflower seeds

1 cup sweetened coconut flakes

½ teaspoon ground cinnamon

¼ teaspoon ground nutmeg

½ teaspoon sea salt

¼ cup canola oil, peanut oil, or coconut oil

¼ cup pure maple syrup

2 tablespoons honey

½ teaspoon pure vanilla extract

1 cup dried fruit, such as raisins, cranberries, or coarsely chopped apricots, cherries, or figs

CALORIES PER SERVING   130
YIELD   8 cups or 16 servings
SERVING SIZE   ½ cup
PREPARATION TIME   10 minutes
TOTAL TIME   40 minutes

BLUEBERRY BANANA OATMEAL

¼ cup fat-free milk

½ cup old-fashioned oats

¼ teaspoon ground cinnamon

½ cup water

2 tablespoons sugar-free maple syrup, or 1 packet sugar substitute

½ banana, sliced

½ cup fresh or frozen blueberries

1 tablespoon chopped toasted walnuts

CALORIES PER SERVING 298

YIELD 1 serving

SERVING SIZE 1 cup

PREPARATION TIME 5 minutes

TOTAL TIME 10 minutes

In a saucepan, combine the milk, oatmeal, cinnamon, and ½ cup water. Bring to a boil over medium-high heat, stirring often to prevent boiling over.

Reduce the heat to medium and simmer until thickened, 3 to 5 minutes.

While the oatmeal is cooking, mash half the banana slices, reserving the remainder for topping. Smash ¼ cup of the blueberries and reserve the remainder for topping.

Add mashed banana and smashed blueberries to oats and stir to combine.

Transfer the oats to a bowl and top with the reserved banana slices and blueberries and the walnuts.

APPLE PIE OATMEAL

In a small saucepan, combine the apple juice, oats, diced apple, raisins, maple syrup, cinnamon, nutmeg, and 1 cup water. Bring to a boil over medium-high heat, stirring often to prevent boiling over.

Reduce the heat to medium and simmer until thickened, 3 to 5 minutes.

Serve in a bowl, topped with the walnuts.

¼ cup apple juice

⅔ cup old-fashioned oats

1 apple, peeled, cored, and diced

2 tablespoons raisins

2 tablespoons sugar-free maple syrup, or 1 packet sugar substitute

¼ teaspoon ground cinnamon

¼ teaspoon ground nutmeg

½ cup water

1 tablespoon chopped toasted walnuts

CALORIES PER SERVING   275

YIELD   2 servings

SERVING SIZE   8 ounces

PREPARATION TIME   5 minutes

TOTAL TIME   10 minutes

PEAR & BLUE CHEESE PITA

¼ cup walnuts, chopped

1 teaspoon balsamic vinegar

1 (6½-inch) whole wheat pita, cut in half to make 2 pockets

1 ounce blue cheese spread

½ pear, cored and sliced

1 cup mixed greens

CALORIES PER SERVING 150

YIELD 1 serving

PREPARATION TIME 5 minutes

TOTAL TIME 10 minutes

Preheat the oven to 250°F.

In a small dry skillet, toast the walnuts over medium-low heat, stirring, until lightly browned and fragrant, 2 to 3 minutes.

Stir in the vinegar in the pan.

Spread the blue cheese in the pita halves.

Fill the pita halves with the pear slices and balsamic walnuts.

Place the pita halves on a baking sheet and toast in the oven for 3 minutes, or until the cheese begins to melt.

Remove from the oven, add the greens, and serve.

CHICKPEA SALAD WITH COUSCOUS AND SPICED CARROTS

In a small saucepan, combine ½ cup water and the salt and bring to a boil. Add the couscous and stir once. Reduce the heat to low, cover, and simmer for 3 minutes. Remove from the heat and let the couscous steam, covered, for 3 minutes. Fluff with a fork. Drain off any liquid remaining in the pan. Transfer the couscous to a serving bowl, stir in 2 teaspoons of the olive oil, cover, and set aside.

In a small dry skillet, toast the cumin, cinnamon, ginger, and cayenne over medium heat until you can smell them, about 1 minute (watch carefully, as spices burn quickly). Add the remaining 2 tablespoons olive oil and cook, stirring, for 1 minute more.

Add the carrots and cook until cooked through but still firm. Remove from the heat and let cool.

Add the cilantro and toss to combine. Set aside.

Stir the canned chickpeas into the couscous.

Add the carrots, cover, and refrigerate for 30 minutes.

Serve the salad topped with the crunchy chickpeas.

¼ teaspoon kosher salt
½ cup couscous
⅛ teaspoon ground cumin
⅛ teaspoon ground cinnamon
⅛ teaspoon ground ginger
    pinch of cayenne pepper
2 teaspoons plus 2 tablespoons extra-virgin olive oil
½ teaspoon minced garlic
¼ teaspoon dried cilantro
1½ cups baby or microwavable carrots
1 cup canned no-salt-added chickpeas, drained and rinsed
2 tablespoons Saffron Road Crunchy Chickpeas

CALORIES PER SERVING 220
YIELD 1 serving
SERVING SIZE 8 ounces
PREPARATION TIME 15 minutes
TOTAL TIME 25 minutes

DEVILED EGG SANDWICH

2 large eggs

2 tablespoons fat-free mayonnaise

1 teaspoon sweet relish

¼ teaspoon yellow mustard

Kosher salt and pepper

⅛ teaspoon smoked paprika

2 slices Nature's Own whole wheat bread

Lettuce leaves and sliced tomato, for serving (optional)

CALORIES PER SERVING 316
YIELD 1 serving
PREPARATION TIME 10 minutes
TOTAL TIME 20 minutes

Place eggs in a medium saucepan and add cold water to cover by 1 inch. Bring the water to a boil over medium heat. Cover, remove from the heat, and let the eggs stand in the hot water for 12 minutes. Drain the eggs in a colander and cool under cold running water. Once cool, peel and chop the eggs and place them in a medium bowl.

Add the mayonnaise, relish, and mustard and stir to combine. Season with salt and pepper. Sprinkle the paprika over the top.

Serve the egg salad on the bread, with lettuce and tomato, if desired.

BONUS MEALS

Here are a few quick meals you may want to try, whether you're following the no-cook plan outlined in chapter 11 or taking the cook-at-home approach. Only the last two require more than 10 minutes of preparation time.

SCRAMBLED EGG (BREAKFAST)

1 large egg, scrambled in a nonstick pan (100 calories)

2 slices whole wheat bread (140 calories)

To drink: ½ cup orange juice (55 calories)

CALORIES PER SERVING 295
PREPARATION TIME 10 minutes

KASHI GOLEAN CRUNCH CEREAL (BREAKFAST)

¾ cup Kashi GOLEAN Crunch (190 calories)

¾ cup fat-free milk (68 calories)

Topped with. ¾ cup fresh blueberries (60 calories)

CALORIES PER SERVING 318
PREPARATION TIME 3 minutes

POST 100% BRAN CEREAL (BREAKFAST)

⅓ cup Post 100% Bran cereal (80 calories)

1 cup fat-free milk (90 calories)

Topped with: ¾ banana, sliced (75 calories)

To drink: ½ cup orange juice (55 calories)

CALORIES PER SERVING 300
PREPARATION TIME 5 minutes

VAN'S 8WG MULTIGRAIN WAFFLES (BREAKFAST)

2 waffles, toasted (180 calories)

Topped with: 1 banana, sliced (100 calories)

CALORIES PER SERVING 280
PREPARATION TIME 6 minutes

SPINACH SALAD (LUNCH)

Combine in an individual serving bowl or on a large plate:

2 cups spinach (14)

½ (5-ounce) can chunk light tuna in water, drained (50)

1 hard-boiled egg (see page 158), diced (100)

2 tablespoons crumbled blue cheese (100)

¼ cup balsamic vinegar (64)

CALORIES PER SERVING 328
PREPARATION TIME 20 minutes

GRILLED MAHIMAHI (LUNCH OR DINNER)

4 ounces mahimahi, grilled (120 calories)

1 cup broccoli florets, sautéed in 1 teaspoon olive oil (70 calories)

1½ slices whole wheat bread, toasted (105 calories)

CALORIES PER SERVING 295
PREPARATION TIME 20 minutes

13

SUPER SMOOTHIES

POWERFUL PUSH-BUTTON NUTRITION

WITH A BLENDER, the correct ingredients, and a few seconds, push a button and you've got a Super Smoothie that can add power to your metabolism.

I was introduced to Super Smoothies by Joe Cirulli, owner of Gainesville Health & Fitness, the largest and most used fitness center in the world. Some six thousand members train there on most days. Cirulli gets up early, goes to bed late, travels extensively, and does not miss a meal or a workout.

For Joe, integrating easy smoothies into his diet was the key to keeping on track. Whether you're dead tired at the end of the day or too lazy to put something together for breakfast, smoothies supply a nutritious, easy-to-digest, non-bloating alternative to a meal.

Smoothie Tips

- Freeze your fruit. Cut the fruit into chunks (leave blueberries and raspberries whole), then lay them out on a tray and freeze until firm. Once frozen, transfer the fruit to zip-lock bags and freeze until ready to use. Frozen fruit helps keep smoothies thick and frosty.

- Use ice in smoothies to give it that thicker, cool, and refreshing texture. But remember, too many ice cubes will make it too thick.
- Make your smoothie thinner by adding coconut water, not fruit juices, which add sugar and calories. Coconut water is rich in potassium and electrolytes.

Purchasing a Blender

Consider these features if you are in the market for a blender.

Easy to store: Consider counter space or cabinet storage, especially if you do not plan to leave it on the countertop.

Power: Since you will be crushing ice and frozen fruit, get a motor with a minimum of 350 watts. Anything less will burn out quickly.

Speed settings: Three different speeds are a good number to help chop your fruit and then blend it smooth.

Jar size: A good blender jar size is at least 40 ounces (5 cups); you could also opt for a personal-size blender. These are great for making single-serving smoothies but frustrating when you want larger amounts.

Ease of cleaning: Look for a blender that does not have to be taken apart to be cleaned.

Durability and warranty: Look for a blender constructed of high-quality materials. Understand that not all warranties are created equal. Be sure to read any warranty as to what it covers and for how long. If the warranty is for the motor, it won't cover a cracked pitcher.

Add Science to the Mix

One research investigation by Lisa M. Davis, published in *Nutrition Journal* in 2010, demonstrated that drinking weight loss shakes as meal replacements does produce positive results. The report found that subjects on a smoothie-shake diet lost an average of more than 12 percent of their body weight during a forty-week period, while subjects on a solid food–based diet lost less than 7 percent.

In another study, published in the *Journal of Nutrition and Metabolism* in 2012, subjects who used one or two meal-replacement shakes daily lost about 2 percent more of their total body weight over a six-month period than subjects who followed diet book suggestions.

In a 2012 report in *Current Nutrition & Food Science*, Joy L. Frestedt and colleagues put a group of obese adults on a plan that replaced breakfast and dinner with nutritious smoothies. There was no exercise requirement and no limit on what else the study participants could eat. After twelve weeks, the subjects had lost up to 18.5 pounds and reported significant improvements in physical and mental health.

Okay, are you ready to make Super Smoothies work for you? Here are seven recipes. Each smoothie makes one serving. One last guideline: Cirulli and I are partial to using a smoothie as breakfast or an afternoon snack. Just make sure the calories are in line with your requirements.

Are You Ready for a Super Smoothie?

All the smoothies that follow make one serving with 300 calories or fewer. For each recipe, combine the ingredients in a high-speed blender, blend until smooth, sip, and enjoy.

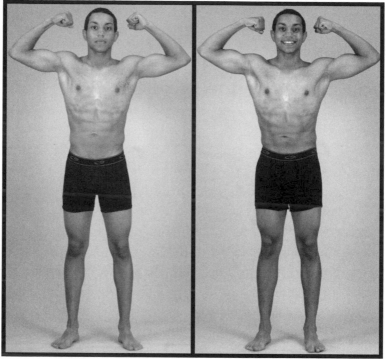

116 pounds   124.25 pounds

GUILLERMO GONZALEZ, age 16, height 5'5"
AFTER 6 WEEKS
(on muscle-building program only)
2 inches added on chest, **1.5** inches on thighs
1.25 inches added on upper arms
8.25 pounds of muscle gain

STRAWBERRY-PISTACHIO PUNCH

½ cup frozen strawberries (24 calories)

¼ avocado (65 calories)

¼ cup pistachios (117 calories)

1 scoop vanilla plant-based protein powder (93 calories)

1 cup green tea, brewed and cold (0 calories)

TOTAL CALORIES 299

DARK CHOCOLATE DELIGHT

2 tablespoons Hershey's Special Dark chocolate syrup (90 calories)

1 frozen banana (100 calories)

1 cup unsweetened almond milk (35 calories)

1 scoop chocolate plant-based protein powder (110 calories)

3 ice cubes

TOTAL CALORIES 335

PEANUT BUTTER–BERRY BLITZ

1 tablespoon peanut butter (94 calories)

10 frozen raspberries (10 calories)

6 frozen blueberries (85 calories)

6 frozen strawberries (24 calories)

½ cup unsweetened almond milk (17 calories)

1 scoop plant-based protein powder (93 calories)

TOTAL CALORIES 323

BANANARAMA

½ cup frozen blueberries (42 calories)

½ frozen banana (50 calories)

2 tablespoons quick-cooking rolled oats (35 calories)

2 teaspoons almonds (22 calories)

½ cup unsweetened almond milk (17 calories)

1 scoop plant-based protein powder (93 calories)

TOTAL CALORIES 259

APPLE A DAY

½ apple (any type), with peel, quartered and cored (49 calories)

¼ frozen banana (17 calories)

½ cup unsweetened almond milk (17 calories)

1 teaspoon flaxseed oil (40 calories)

3 or 4 dashes of ground cinnamon

2 or 3 dashes of ground nutmeg

2 or 3 dashes of ground ginger

1 scoop vanilla plant-based protein powder (93 calories)

TOTAL CALORIES 216

PURPLE HEAVEN

½ cup frozen blueberries (42 calories)

1½ teaspoons almond butter (51 calories)

½ cup unsweetened almond milk (17 calories)

1 scoop vanilla plant-based protein powder (93 calories)

3 ice cubes

TOTAL CALORIES 203

AVOCADO GO GO

¼ avocado (40 calories)

½ frozen banana (34 calories)

½ cup frozen blueberries (42 calories)

½ cup unsweetened almond milk (17 calories)

1 scoop chocolate plant-based protein powder (110 calories)

TOTAL CALORIES 243

Prepare and Adapt

Multiple studies show that adding a smoothie to your fat-loss eating plan can result in greater fat loss. Why? Because blender shakes are simple, fast, nutritious, and almost perfect meal replacements. Many of the most successful Killing Fat participants had a smoothie almost daily for breakfast or lunch.

Learn from Joe Cirulli's advice: *Prepare and adapt.* You can easily add or subtract ingredients from each of the smoothie recipes. Just keep each one in the 300-calorie range and you'll be well on your way to push-button fat-loss success.

Smoothies and Muscle Building for Teenagers

For many bodybuilders and young guys trying to gain muscle, smoothies and blender drinks are a regular part of their nutritional plan. Joe Cirulli and I have both applied them successfully throughout our careers. These types of smoothies, however, contain a lot more calories than the 300 calories suggested above.

I've encouraged many of my teenage trainees, such as Jordan Rapport and Chris Medary (see chapter 3), to consume smoothies as part of their meal plans to get bigger and stronger. Cirulli has done the same in working with teenagers in Gainesville.

Each summer at Gainesville Health & Fitness, Cirulli allows hundreds of teenagers to use the strength-training facilities during the midmornings at no charge. Most of the supervision is directed by the club's floor instructors.

One such floor instructor, who worked with many teenagers successfully in 2012, was Guillermo Gonzalez, age eighteen. Gonzalez not only guided these young people, but took it upon himself to add muscle to his own physique. The before-and-after photographs on page 184 show that his work paid off. Gonzalez often used various smoothies, which are available at Gainesville Health & Fitness, and mastered the thermodynamic synergy concepts I've discussed in this book to achieve his muscle-building goals.

Another teenager, Will Wright (page 188), a trainee of mine from Orlando, was also a fan of smoothies. He noted a more gradual muscle-building progression than Gonzalez did. Wright trained approximately once a week for fifty weeks and gained 24.5 pounds of muscle. That muscle helped him play championship football for Windermere Prep in Orlando during 2014 and 2015.

Wright has continued with his training and is now 6 feet 4 inches tall and weighs 220 pounds. He enrolled at Florida State University in the fall of 2018.

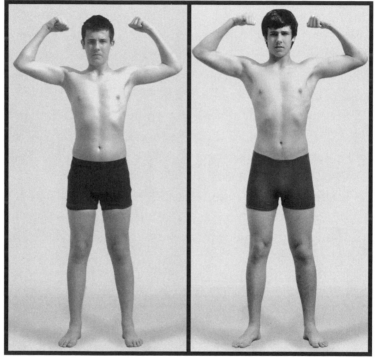

149.5 pounds   **174** pounds

WILL WRIGHT, age 15, height 5'10"
AFTER 12 MONTHS
(on muscle-building program only)
4.5 inches added to chest
2.125 inches added to arms, **3** inches on thighs
24.5 pounds of muscle gain

14

MEAL PLANS

DAYS 1 TO 7 AND
DAYS 8 TO 14

DIETERS OFTEN NEED help in planning a series of meals that are not only tasty and filling, but also keep their enthusiasm at high levels. Chef Billie DeNunzio and I have taught hundreds of people how to organize low-calorie meals efficiently. Our guidelines are as follows:

- First, in your diet, note the meals per day and the calories per meal.
- Second, make a list of all the appropriate foods and recipes for breakfast, lunch, dinner, and snacks.
- Third, combine the meals with the selected foods and recipes into a table for easy planning and preparation.

Killing Fat Meals and Daily Calorie Guidelines

The Killing Fat meals are small and evenly spaced throughout the day.

During weeks 1 and 2, the total calories per day are 1,400 for women and 1,600 for men.

Below are the calorie counts of the six small meals for each day:

1. Breakfast: 300 calories
2. Midmorning snack: 100 calories
3. Lunch: 300 calories for women, 400 calories for men
4. Afternoon snack: 200 calories
5. Dinner: 300 calories for women, 400 calories for men
6. Evening snack: 200 calories

Meal Plan, Days 1 to 7

On page 191 is the Killing Fat meal plan for days 1 to 7, which notes a recipe, food, or combination of foods for the required calories at the specified time of day. The foods listed are only suggestions; you can mix and match as you like, as long as you stay within daily calorie parameters.

Meal Plan, Days 8 to 14

The meal plan for days 8 to 14 (page 192) is similar to the plan for days 1 to 7. Once again, the foods and recipes listed are only suggestions—follow them closely or make changes as you like. Just remember to keep your calories at the same approximate number per meal and total overall for the day.

MEAL PLAN DAYS 1 TO 7

	DAY 1	DAY 2	DAY 3	DAY 4	DAY 5	DAY 6	DAY 7
BREAKFAST 300 calories	Scrambled Egg (p. 179), 295 cal	Homemade Granola Cereal (p. 173), 295 cal	Whole Wheat Bagel (p. 147), 300 cal	Multigrain Waffles (p. 180), 280 cal	Blueberry Banana Oatmeal (p. 174), 298 cal	Egg White Omelet (p. 172), 304 cal	Homemade Granola Cereal (p. 173), 295 cal
SNACK 100 calories	14 almonds, 100 cal	1 cup low-fat or fat-free yogurt, 100 cal	1 apple, 100 cal	1 Cottage Doubles, 100 cal	1 ounce raisins, 82 cal	14 cashews, 100 cal	½ cantaloupe, 94 cal
LUNCH 300 calories Men: Add 100 calories (see p. 148)	Turkey Sandwich (p. 148), 300 cal	Peanut Butter–Berry Blitz (p. 185), 323 cal	Spinach Salad (p. 180) 315 cal	Deviled Egg Sandwich (p. 178), 316 cal	Shake (p. 147), 295 cal	Ham Sandwich (p. 148), 300 cal	Tuna Salad with Corn & Peas (p. 151), 260 cal
SNACK 200 calories	1 cup low-fat or fat-free yogurt, 100 cal and 1 ounce raisins, 82 cal	1 apple, 100 cal and 14 cashews, 100 cal	½ cantaloupe 94 cal and 14 almonds, 100 cal	2 cups light popcorn, 100 cal and 1 cup low-fat or fat-free yogurt, 100 cal	14 cashews, 100 cal and 5 prunes, 100 cal	2 cups light popcorn, 100 cal and 14 almonds, 100 cal	1 apple, 100 cal and 1 Cottage Doubles, 100 cal
DINNER 300 calories Men: Add 100 calories (see page 149)	Robust Turkey Meatball Soup, (p. 156), 246 cal	Rosemary Roasted Chicken (p. 170), 332 cal	Quick Veggie Mock Chicken (p. 163), 310 cal	Black Bean Veggie Patties (p. 155), 300 cal	Five-Cheese Lasagna (Michelina's), 270 cal	Zesty Lime Shrimp Salad (p. 162), 300 cal	Thai Beef Salad (p. 160), 301 cal
SNACK 200 calories	2 cups light popcorn, 100 cal and 1 ounce raisins, 82 cal	1 cup low-fat or fat-free yogurt, 100 cal and 14 almonds, 100 cal	5 prunes, 100 cal and 1 Cottage Doubles, 100 cal	½ cantaloupe, 94 cal and 1 cup low-fat or fat-free yogurt, 100 cal	1 apple, 100 cal and 14 almonds, 100 cal	4 cups light popcorn, 200 cal	14 cashews, 100 cal and 1 ounce raisins, 82 cal

MEAL PLAN DAYS 8 TO 14

	DAY 8	DAY 9	DAY 10	DAY 11	DAY 12	DAY 13	DAY 14
BREAKFAST 300 calories	Apple Pie Oatmeal (p. 175), 275 cal	Scrambled Egg (p. 179), 295 cal	Post 100% Bran Cereal (p. 179), 300 cal	Whole wheat bagel (p. 147), 300 cal	Smoothie: Strawberry-Pistachio Punch (p. 184), 299 cal	English muffin and hard-boiled egg (p. 147), 298 cal	Egg White Omelet (p. 172), 304 cal
SNACK 100 calories	1 cup low-fat or fat-free yogurt, 100 cal	1 ounce raisins, 82 cal	1 Cottage Doubles, 100 cal	½ cantaloupe, 94 cal	14 cashews, 100 cal	1 apple, 100 cal	5 prunes, 100 cal
LUNCH 300 calories Men: Add 100 calories (see p. 148)	Pear & Blue Cheese Pita (p. 176), 190 cal	Chickpea Salad with Spiced Carrots (p. 177), 290 cal	Black Bean with Red Quinoa Soup (Campbell's Well Yes!), 280 cal	Turkey Sandwich (p. 148), 300 cal	Tuna-Bean Salad (p. 151), 267 cal	Spinach Salad (p. 180), 315 cal	Grilled Mahimahi (p. 180), 295 cal
SNACK 200 calories	1 Cottage Doubles, 100 cal and 14 almonds, 100 cal	4 cups light popcorn, 200 cal	1 apple, 100 cal and 1 cup low-fat or fat-free yogurt, 100 cal	14 cashews, 100 cal and 1 ounce raisins, 82 cal	½ cantaloupe, 94 cal and 5 prunes, 100 cal	1 apple, 100 cal and 14 almonds, 100 cal	1 cup low-fat or fat-free yogurt, 100 cal and 1 ounce raisins, 82 cal
DINNER 300 calories Men: Add 100 calories (see p. 149)	Quinoa Pilaf with Pistachios (p. 157), 283 cal	Spaghetti Squash Turkey Bolognese (p. 168), 301 cal	Cobb Salad with Turkey Cutlets (p. 158), 360 cal	Grilled Mahimahi (p. 180), 295 cal	Quick Veggie Mock Chicken (p. 166), 310 cal	Skirt Steak Salad (p. 171), 284 cal for 2 cups (women) 425 cal for 3 cups (men)	Zesty Lime Shrimp Salad (p. 162), 300 cal
SNACK 200 calories	1 Cottage Doubles, 100 cal and 14 cashews, 100 cal	1 apple, 100 cal and 1 ounce raisins, 82 cal	14 almonds, 100 cal and 1 cup low-fat or fat-free yogurt, 100 cal	½ cantaloupe, 94 cal and 1 ounce raisins, 82 cal	2 cups light popcorn, 100 cal and 1 cup low-fat or fat-free yogurt, 100 cal	14 cashews, 100 cal and 1 cup low-fat or fat-free yogurt, 100 cal	5 prunes, 100 cal and 1 Cottage Doubles, 100 cal

Reminder: Lower Calorie Intake During Weeks 3 and 4 and Weeks 5 and 6

The daily calorie intake declines by 100 calories for both women and men before weeks 3 and 4. And there's another 100-calorie decrease before weeks 5 and 6. Women go from 1,400 to 1,300 to 1,200 calories. Men move from 1,600 to 1,500 to 1,400 calories. This descending-calorie plan keeps the metabolism on a more even keel.

To accomplish this, the size of your main meals remains unchanged, but you eliminate one Afternoon Snack (–100 calories) for weeks 3 and 4, and one Evening Snack (–100 calories) at the start of weeks 5 and 6. In other words, only the number of snacks is decreased. As you progress through the six-week program, you should modify your snack tables accordingly.

Organize and Move Forward

The meal plans for Days 1 to 7 and Days 8 to 14 allow you to manage your food in advance, which will keep you in the driver's seat to achieve significant fat loss. Meaningful preparation is required, but the results will be well worth the effort.

15

POSITIVE RESULTS FROM NEGATIVE ROUTINES

MUSCLE BUILDING FOR WEEKS 1 TO 6

JUST ABOUT EVERY weight loss expert says you can't lose fat and build muscle at the same time. Their emphasis on exercise is usually an elevated-heart-rate routine, stretching for flexibility, or a long walking visit with a couple of friends. In other words, their exercise routines are more of a recreational endeavor than a body-transforming workout.

Of course, these experts have never experienced proper strength training—and especially not negative-accentuated 30–10–30 training.

The Physics of the Negative

Research with positive and negative effort reveals that strength training obeys the basic physical laws described centuries ago by Isaac Newton. Newton's law of inertia states that an object at rest tends to stay at rest unless acted upon by an outside force. This applies directly to the lifting of a weight at the start of a concentric (positive) muscle action.

For example, in the standing barbell curl, the weight begins at rest with the biceps muscle ready to act. If the muscular force exceeds the inertia of the barbell, movement occurs and the barbell is lifted. Concentric (positive) muscle action, therefore, is used to initiate, maintain, or increase motion of an object.

An eccentric (negative) muscle action has a different effect. In Newton's law of acceleration, an object in motion tends to stay in motion unless acted upon by an outside force. In strength training, an object that has been raised by concentric (positive) muscle action is now pulled back by the force of gravity. Only by muscular force being exerted against the descending weight can it be prevented from accelerating downward.

Positive and negative muscle actions have evolved to accommodate the laws of motion. Muscle force during shortening is less than force during lengthening because it is harder to create a new bond than to break an existing one.

The process of shortening is complex, energy dependent, and based on creating new chemical bonds. But once formed, these bonds are extremely stable and thus make the lengthening process so appropriate for overloading. That's why a person can become stronger *quickly* with heavy negative resistance lowered slowly.

In other words, the stability of the existing chemical bonds involved in lowering a heavy resistance reacts appropriately and adapts well to the right negative-accentuated training, combined with more-than-adequate rest and sleep.

Ten Reasons to Accentuate the Negative

After reviewing the scientific literature on positive and negative exercise, I've concluded that negative training:

- Involves a heavier-than-normal overload—which means more force output and more muscle fibers recruited.
- Recruits more fast-twitch muscle fibers—which contribute predominantly to muscular size.
- Ensures a higher level of stress per motor unit—which supplies greater stimulation of the involved muscle fibers.
- Requires greater neural adaptation—which reinforces cross-education of strength gains from one limb or side to the other.
- Causes more microscopic muscle fiber tears—which ignite the muscle-building process.
- Works the entire joint structure—which results in more strength, stability, range of motion, and healing properties.
- Applies well to postsurgical therapy—which is advantageous in rehabilitation.
- Maintains strength gains longer—which counter the detraining process.
- Transfers strength gains to positive work—which is valuable in lifting performance.
- Allows for greater work in less time—which means more efficient training sessions and faster results.

One More In-Depth Reason to Accentuate the Negative

This last reason may, in fact, be the most important reason of all. This concept relates directly to my negative-accentuated studies in Gainesville.

Negative training makes a deeper muscular inroad, repetition by repetition, throughout the entire set—which stimulates the production of growth hormone (GH), insulin-like growth factor 1 (IGF-1), mechano growth factor (MGF), interleukin-6 (IL-6), and interleukin-15 (IL-15).

GH, IGF-1, MGF, IL-6, and IL-15 pulsating into the bloodstream not only lead to muscle hypertrophy, but also oxidize fat cell content at a faster-than-normal rate.

Releasing fat rapidly is probably assisted by a related hormone's anabolic influence on both muscle and fat. That hormone is insulin. Apparently, intense negative-accentuated training *decreases* the effect of insulin on fat and *increases* the effect of insulin on muscle.

In other words, with negative-accentuated training, the deeper muscular inroad diminishes fat cells' insulin sensitivity, and those cells begin to shrink. As insulin sensitivity in the muscle elevates, glucose and nutrients are directed preferentially into muscle cells, which expand.

Expanded muscle cells and shrunken fat cells equal more muscle and less fat. More muscle and less fat equal a stronger, leaner, better-shaped body. Negative-accentuated training, by stimulating and directing the body's natural hormones, provides the best possible way to build muscle and lose fat *quickly*.

Before I get into the three phases of the Killing Fat negative-training routines, let's review the points you'll be practicing.

Appropriate Actions for Negative Training

Examine first: Spend several minutes looking over the exercises listed in the various routines in this chapter. Each exercise is detailed and illustrated in chapter 9, so you'll want to refer back to them frequently.

Choose between free-weight movements and machine exercises: If you train at home, you may want to apply free-weight movements. If you belong to a commercial fitness center or gym, you'll probably have access to machines. Most of the men and women involved in the Killing Fat research used machine exercises. You could also do a mix of both.

Select the appropriate resistance: Initially, it's important that you learn how to perform each recommended exercise correctly. You'll learn better if the resistance is neither too heavy nor too light. Try to select a moderate resistance at first, something you can do easily for 20–10–20: a 20-second negative; 10 positive-negative repetitions in a normal manner; and a final 20-second negative. After the first week, increase the 20-second intervals to 30 seconds, and increase the resistance so the 30–10–30 is challenging.

Control your movements: Rushing each exercise diminishes results and can cause injury. Have a watch with a second hand (or, better yet, a big clock) in plain sight, or have a spotter help with the counting, to keep your deliberate negatives at the called-for number.

Count the seconds of each stroke: Start by aiming for 20 to 30 seconds on each negative and record the actual number of seconds you hit for each negative phase. When you can do the complete 30–10–30, increase the resistance by 5 percent at your next workout and continue this progression throughout the program.

Expect some soreness: Soreness in exercised body parts is an indication that you've stretched and contracted little-used muscles. Expect some soreness after each of your workouts, especially the ones that involve new exercises. Soreness is usually in the muscle. Pain, however, occurs in the joints and connective tissues. As you become accustomed to negative-accentuated training, you'll start understanding the differences between the two. Soreness is good; pain is not.

Decrease your frequency: The idea is to do less as you get stronger. The frequency of training during weeks 1 through 6 is twice a week, which usually means a training session on Monday and Thursday, or Tuesday and Friday. After six weeks, depending on your progress, you may reduce your training to three times every two weeks. Eventually, you may choose to train only once a week.

Each training session involves one set each of six to ten exercises. Each 30–10–30 exercise requires approximately 60 to 90 seconds. Moving from one exercise to the next takes about 60 seconds. So each routine can be performed in 25 minutes or less. The next section includes routines for free weights, machines, and both combined.

Free-Weight Routines

Free-weight routines are primarily performed with barbells and dumbbells, as well as a bench and support racks. An asterisk (*) indicates an exercise added to the previous week's routine.

WEEKS 1 AND 2

Dumbbell Squat (page 87)

Barbell Bench Press (page 90)

Barbell Curl (page 93)

Barbell Overhead Press (page 97)

Dumbbell Triceps Extension (page 100)

Sit-Up on Declined Board (page 102)

WEEKS 3 AND 4

Dumbbell Squat (page 87)

Barbell Bench Press (page 90)

Barbell Curl (page 93)

Barbell Overhead Press (page 97)

Dumbbell Triceps Extension (page 100)

Negative-Only Chin-Up* (page 107)

Negative-Only Dip* (page 105)

Sit-Up on Declined Board (page 102)

WEEKS 5 AND 6

Dumbbell Squat (page 87)

Barbell Bench Press (page 90)

Barbell Curl (page 93)

Barbell Overhead Press (page 97)

Dumbbell Triceps Extension (page 100)

Negative-Only Chin-Up (page 107)

Negative-Only Dip (page 105)

Dumbbell Hammer Curl* (page 95)

Barbell Squat* (page 84)

Sit-Up on Declined Board (page 102)

Machine Routines

For these routines, you'll need access to some basic strength-training machines—such as Nautilus, Cybex, Life Fitness, MedX, Hammer Strength, or Body-Solid—which are found in fitness centers throughout the United States and Canada. Where there is a choice, alternate between them or use one or the other. Be sure to keep accurate records of your selections and progress. An asterisk (*) indicates an exercise added to the previous week's routine.

WEEKS 1 AND 2

Leg Curl (page 112)

Leg Press (page 115)

Chest Press (page 121)

Pulldown on Lat Machine (page 123)

Barbell Overhead Press (page 97)

Abdominal Crunch (page 127)

WEEKS 3 AND 4

Leg Curl (page 112)

Leg Extension* (page 109)

Leg Press (page 115)

Chest Press (page 121)

Pulldown on Lat Machine (page 123)

Overhead Press (page 97)

Barbell Curl* (page 93)

Abdominal Crunch (page 127)

WEEKS 5 AND 6

Leg Curl (page 112)

Leg Extension (page 109)

Leg Press (page 115)

Calf Raise (standing)* (page 118)

Chest Press (page 121)

Pulldown on Lat Machine (page 123)

Barbell Overhead Press (page 97)

Barbell Curl (page 93)

Pushdown on Lat Machine* (page 125)

Abdominal Crunch (page 127)

Combination Machine/ Free-Weight Routines

These routines involve an advanced technique called pre-exhaustion, where two exercises are performed back to back, with minimum rest in between. Properly applied, you'll feel them deep within the involved muscles.

WEEKS 1 AND 2

Leg Extension (page 109), immediately followed by Leg Press (page 115)

Leg Curl (page 112), immediately followed by Dumbbell Squat (page 87)

Chest Press (page 121)

Pulldown on Lat Machine (page 123)

WEEKS 3 AND 4

Leg Extension (page 109), immediately followed by Leg Press (page 115)

Dumbbell Hammer Curl (page 95), immediately followed by Negative-Only Chin-Up (page 107)

Pushdown on Lat Machine (page 125), immediately followed by Negative-Only Dip (page 105)

Calf Raise (standing) (page 118)

Sit-Up on Declined Board (page 102)

WEEKS 5 AND 6

Leg Curl (page 112), immediately followed by Dumbbell Squat (page 87)

Barbell Overhead Press (page 97), immediately followed by Negative-Only Dip (page 105)

Pulldown on Lat Machine (page 123), immediately followed by Negative-Only Chin-Up (page 107)

Pushdown on Lat Machine (page 125), immediately followed by Chest Press (page 121)

Barbell Curl (page 93)

Abdominal Crunch (page 127)

Firemen Fight Fat with Fire

In the United States, there are more than 1,100,000 firefighters serving 30,145 fire departments and 55,400 fire stations. I live in Orlando, Florida. In Orange County, which surrounds the city, there are 58 fire

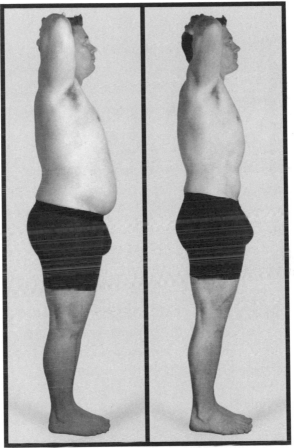

283 pounds   243 pounds
TOM O'CONNELL, age 43, height 6'1"
AFTER 10 WEEKS
47.6 pounds of fat loss
8.25 inches off waist
7.6 pounds of muscle gain

stations. According to Tom O'Connell, who has been a fireman in Orlando for thirteen years, 70 percent of the Orange County firemen are overfat.

"We are all big eaters and drinkers," O'Connell said, "and it shows on our bodies. But many of us regularly lift weights, and we're a strong bunch—because we have to use our strength every week." O'Connell is talking about the pulling, pushing, and carrying operations that are required each day in their emergency responding.

"My firefighting team," O'Connell continued, "knows we need to get rid of some fat . . . and we want you to help us."

I'd been telling O'Connell about my new 30–10–30, negative-accentuated technique and my Killing Fat diet, and he'd received permission for me to talk about these programs to interested men in his unit.

Twelve firefighters from Fire Station #54, near SeaWorld Orlando, volunteered in August 2016 to participate in my Killing Fat program. By my standards, each man was overfat. My goal was for the group to do the Killing Fat program exactly as stated in this book. Unfortunately, Hurricane Matthew's destruction in central Florida in September 2016 interrupted the program, and I had to shorten the first six weeks to four weeks.

All the firefighters were tested before the start of the program and again four weeks later at its conclusion. Of the twelve men who started the program, one dropped out; the remaining eleven men completed four weeks of the Killing Fat program. Their starting averages were as follows:

Age: 40.8 years
Height: 70.6 inches
Weight: 238.6 pounds
Waist: 44.21 inches

At the end of four weeks, their average results were as follows:

Fat loss: 20.18 pounds

Muscle gain: 4.1 pounds

Waist drop: 4.5 inches

The top losers of fat were Thomas O'Connell at 32.72 pounds, James Thacker at 26.06 pounds, and Garrett Wienckowski at 22.36 pounds.

Of the eleven finishers, five men were satisfied with their results after four weeks, and six decided to continue the program for another six weeks; one subsequently dropped out. Things progressed nicely, and after six weeks, the averages for the five firemen for the combined ten weeks of the program were:

Fat loss: 36.73 pounds

Muscle gain: 5.69 pounds

Waist drop: 6.875 inches

Again, the top fat-losers were O'Connell at 47.6 pounds, Thacker at 38.73 pounds, and Wienckowski at 33.84 pounds. O'Connell also trimmed 9.25 inches off his waist.

In conclusion, the firefighters' averages for both four weeks and ten weeks were near the highest average numbers I've achieved in fat transfer for those time periods. Killing Fat with thermodynamic synergy worked big-time for the firefighters . . . and it will for you, too.

Remember what the firemen in Orlando learned:

You can fight fat with fire.

16

MORE FAT LOSS
WEEKS 7 THROUGH 12

FOR THE FIRST time in my life, I can dunk a basketball with both hands," said twenty-two-year-old Doug Spratt to me back in 1984. "I could never do that in high school or college."

Spratt was attending a Nautilus Training Seminar in Florida. He had a degree in exercise science and was detailing how he had successfully lost 25 pounds of fat and built 10 pounds of muscle . . . at a Nautilus club in St. Joseph, Missouri. At 6 feet 4 inches tall with a body weight of 185 pounds, Spratt was in ripped condition.

In 1990, I ran into Spratt again at a Nautilus facility in Merritt Island, Florida, where he was working. I had just published my book *The Nautilus Diet*, and his club was involved in a version of that diet. Eventually, Spratt opened his own club, Body Coach, in Orlando.

When I moved from Gainesville to Orlando in 1998, Spratt was one of the first people I contacted. I needed a place to train, and I knew he had the necessary equipment. Spratt also had his dietary information up to date, and he always seemed to be working with several young men and women who needed to remove fat. With some of those Body Coach members, it was like Spratt specialized in long-term fat loss: getting people over the initial six-week period and supervising them through twelve, eighteen, and even twenty-four weeks of fat loss.

One person Spratt trained with success was his sister, Allison.

Allison Spratt: "Life Was Passing Me By"

"I used to be a compulsive eater," Allison told me. "Sometimes I'd go all day without food. Then, after work, I'd eat almost continuously from six p.m. to eleven p.m. If that wasn't enough, on my really stressed-out days, I'd snack on high-calorie foods in the mornings and in the afternoons. As you can imagine, my body weight soared. At the same time, my self-image sunk to an all-time low.

"I had a real dilemma. If I stayed home at night, I'd eat. If I went out, I was embarrassed about the way I looked. I felt less and less in control and very much alone. It just seemed like life was passing me by.

"'Help,' I kept saying to myself. 'Somebody, please help me!'"

Allison Accepts Doug's Challenge

"It was the Christmas of 1997," Allison remembered, "and my brother, Doug, responded to my pleas. He listened sincerely to all my problems. He then invited me to relocate to Florida, where he had his Body Coach fitness center. He advised me to avoid all the highly advertised weight loss gimmicks and then challenged me to get involved in a scientific fat-loss program. Knowing Doug would be there to provide supervision, I accepted his challenge.

"Doug has long been a believer in Ellington Darden's books. Thus, he started me reading and applying the guidelines in *The Nautilus Diet* and *A Flat Stomach ASAP.*

"After twelve weeks," Allison said, smiling, "I had to buy new clothes. After two more six-week sessions, or a total of twenty-four weeks, all my new clothes were too loose. After another six-week session, and me lighter by seventy pounds of fat, Doug invited Ellington over to watch me train. He commented about my strength, form, and focus. It was such a treat when, just eight months earlier, I would have hidden in the dressing room during his entire visit.

"A couple of hours later, Doug took some pictures of Ellington and me together. I was so happy."

Getting Even . . . And Liking It!

"My life has changed so much for the better," Allison said. "Eight months ago, I was despondent and distraught about my body and many of my habits. It seemed like life had a grudge against me. With the right direction and discipline, I got even—I got even by conquering the underlying causes, such as large meals and a lack of intense exercise.

"And you know what? My body rewarded me for it. Now I'm in charge of my own life."

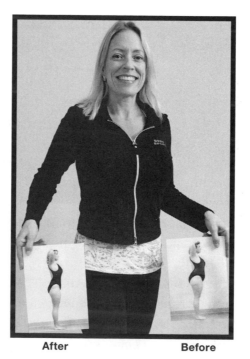

After   Before

Allison Spratt lost 70 pounds in 1998 and it changed
her life. Twenty years later (above) and she has
not regained even 1 pound of fat.

Allison Spratt: Twenty Years Later

Here's what Allison said in early 2018: "Doug recently took my measurements, and he says my body fat percentage has gone from twenty-four to eighteen. I weighed 142.5 pounds in 1998 and I weigh exactly the same 142.5 today. That means that over twenty years, I've lost an additional 8.55 pounds of fat and—get this—I've built 8.55 pounds of muscle.

"I want Doug to share some of his amazing dietary guides, which I've successfully applied for more than twenty years. Not only will they help you for six weeks, twelve weeks, or until you kill your excessive fat—they'll become useful to you for years and years in the future."

DOUG SPRATT TALKS FAT LOSS

Losing body fat requires extra discipline, motivation, and patience. Understanding how the process works is half the battle. The main thing you need to realize is that you will lose body fat in the reverse order you gained it, meaning the first place you gained it is going to be the last place you lose it. This is genetically determined, and no matter what kind of exercises you are doing, you will still lose fat the exact same way.

POWERFUL GENETICS

Genetics determine how tall you will be, how big your feet will be, your eye and hair color, even the potential of how fast you can run, how high you can jump, how big your muscles can get, and of course where and how fat will come off the body.

The first place women gain fat is usually in the hips or thighs; for men, it's usually around the navel area or the sides of the waist (those "love handles"). There are exceptions to this, but once again, it's in your family history. The last places you gain fat are usually the face, chin, hands, and feet. Therefore, this is the first place you will notice it coming off, so be patient and stay on track, and soon you will notice the fat coming off the areas you want it to.

BODY RESHAPING

Reshaping and building your body requires practice. Practice and repetition are what you need to progress. Overlearning is the key to getting and maintaining results.

The best thing to do if you fall off the wagon is not worry about it. You are going to make mistakes. The key is to learn from your mistakes.

Practice, practice, practice. Plan, plan, plan. Learn from your "off" moments. Anticipate them.

Most of all, do not ever give up. Remember, it is just food. You control it. It does not control you.

FOCUS ON FIBER

A fiber-rich diet can help prevent cancer, diabetes, obesity, and heart disease. It also makes you feel fuller! Fiber may also reduce blood pressure and bad cholesterol. Research has shown that dietary fiber can help prevent colon cancer. Colon cancer is the number two most fatal, second only to lung cancer. An estimated 65,000 Americans die from it every year. The average American eats less than 12 grams of fiber a day; try to work your way up to 20 to 25 grams a day. *Important:* Make sure you increase the amount of fiber you take in slowly, and increase your water intake at the same time.

There are two basic classifications of fiber: soluble and insoluble. Each has its own function and benefits, so it's best to try to get a mix of both instead of all one kind.

Insoluble fiber will not dissolve in water, so it moves through the body very quickly, taking whatever is around it with it. It's also known as "nature's broom."

Soluble fiber dissolves in water, and in the body it turns into a thick viscous gel that moves through the digestive tract very slowly. Therefore, if you eat a food high in soluble fiber, you'll feel fuller longer, so you are going to eat less. Soluble fiber also slows the absorption rate of glucose in the body, so it will help you avoid blood sugar highs and lows. What's more, it inhibits the reabsorption of bile into the system, so your liver is going to have to get its cholesterol fix from your blood, which means your blood serum cholesterol is going to go down.

The best fiber choices include:

- Fresh vegetables (raw, steamed, grilled)
- Most whole fresh fruits
- Nuts and seeds
- Beans, peas, and lentils

DOUG AND ALLISON'S BEST ADVICE FOR KILLING FAT

- Build muscle. Muscle is the fountain of youth.
- Emphasize superhydration and staying cool. Always have your insulated water bottle with you.
- Brush and floss your teeth. If you crave certain foods, try brushing your teeth and tongue. It is harder to eat with a clean, minty taste in your mouth.
- Cut back on your evening TV. Watching television can hypnotize you to the point where you snack and do not realize how much you have eaten. Make a personal rule to never eat while watching TV.
- Get extra sleep and rest. This is probably the most important rule of all, because sleep facilitates both fat loss and muscle recovery.
- Stay busy. Do activities that will keep your mind preoccupied and off food.

- Eat plenty of green vegetables. Vegetables fill you up at a cost of fewer calories and fat grams.

- Become a professional label reader. Pay attention not only to calories but also to trans fat, sodium, and vitamin content.

- Cut back on alcohol. Not only is alcohol high in calories, but it interferes with kidney function, which inhibits the efficiency of your body's purification systems. That means your body cannot burn fat efficiently.

- Keep a diary of your food intake and physical activity. Doing so will help you master your daily lifestyle.

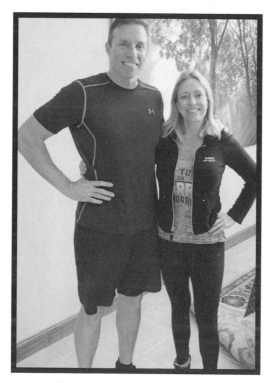

Brother and sister, Doug Spratt, age 56, and Allison Spratt, age 46, are personal trainers. Doug is in Orlando and Allison works out of St. Joseph, Missouri.

Dietary Directions, Weeks 7 Through 12

In terms of diet, the instructions for weeks 7 through 12 are simple: Repeat what you've been doing for the last six weeks in almost the same way for another six weeks.

I've had some people who needed to lose 100 pounds or more go through the six-week eating plan five consecutive times. That's 6 weeks x 5 = 30 weeks of the same basic foods.

There is some variation among foods—from three to five choices each for breakfast, lunch, dinner, and snacks—so the entire plan is certainly doable for at least six months. If you like to cook, there are at least 20 recipes in chapter 12, any of which are ready to join in the action.

Negative-Accentuated Training, Weeks 7 Through 12

During weeks 5 and 6, you performed one set each of ten exercises . . . and you repeated the routine progressively twice a week. I want you to continue with this routine of ten exercises twice a week until you lose your excess fat.

Your negative-accentuated goal is to double your strength in all your basic exercises. If you did 100 pounds on the chest press machine for 30–10–30 when you started, then your goal is to work up to 200 pounds for 30–10–30. Many guys can reach that goal on the basic exercises within four to six months.

Eventually, to continue to build strength, you'll need to reduce the frequency of your training from twice a week to three times in two weeks.

Your other practices—such as superhydration and extra sleeping—should remain unchanged.

To close this chapter, Doug Spratt said it best:

"Muscle is the fountain of youth."

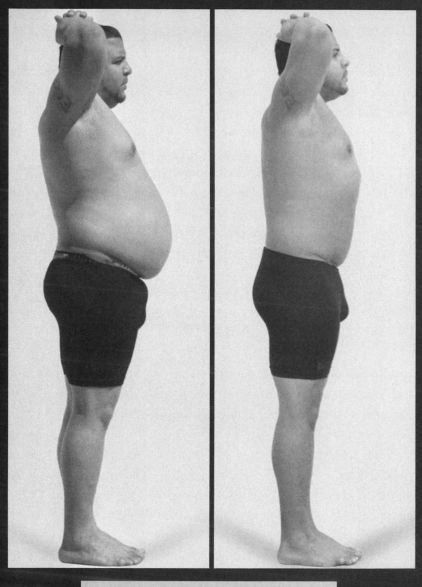

253.5 pounds   **214.5** pounds

EDGARDO RIVERA, age 29, height 5'9"
AFTER 12 WEEKS
50.78 pounds of fat loss
9.875 inches off waist
11.78 pounds of muscle gain

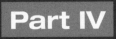
Part IV

SPECIFIC THERMO-DYNAMIC TACTICS

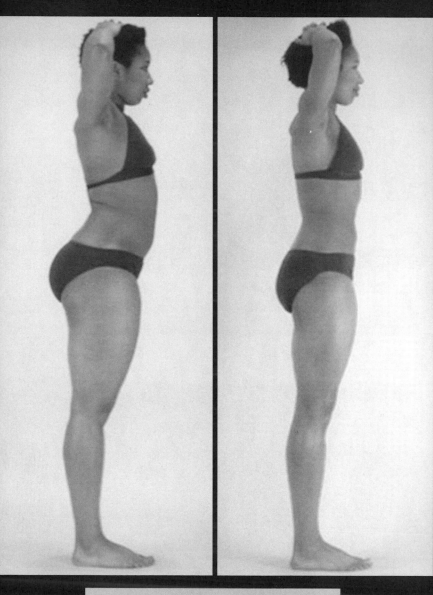

154.6 pounds   130.6 pounds

CANDACE SPENCER, age 21, height 5'5"
AFTER 12 WEEKS
28.27 pounds of fat loss
5.5 inches off waist, **7** inches off hips
4.27 pounds of muscle gain

17

ICE-COLD DRINKING WATER

A COOL WAY TO BURN FAT

TED TUCKER, AGE thirty-eight, was almost ready to begin my Killing Fat program. He definitely needed to get rid of at least 40 pounds of fat, and I had just told him that one of my requirements was he must drink 1 gallon of ice-cold water a day.

"I'm a cartoonist," Tucker said, "and I'm in and out of the Orlando theme parks all day directing my team of artists. I can't imagine having to carry that water bottle, maybe two of them, with me everywhere I go."

"Yes, Ted," I replied, "and that's easy to do with a simple shoulder strap or backpack. It's really no big deal."

"But then, if a gallon goes in, doesn't a gallon have to come out?" Tucker asked. "Then I'll have to search for restrooms all over the place," he noted, answering his own question.

"Ted, you already know that the large theme parks probably operate the cleanest restrooms in the world," I said. "And they are located appropriately throughout the parks. You will never have to hold it or wait in line."

"Let me think about it a little more," Tucker replied. I could tell by his tone that he was bending a little.

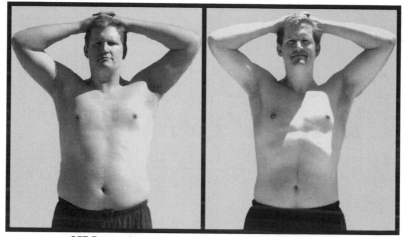

257.5 pounds   **220.12** pounds

TED TUCKER, age 38, height 6'4.5"
AFTER 10 WEEKS
41.38 pounds of fat loss
6.625 inches off waist
4 pounds of muscle gain

"Ted, I want you to give the water drinking a try for at least a week, along with the other requirements," I continued. "One week . . . and let's see how it goes."

"One week." Tucker nodded. "Okay, I'll give it a try . . . for seven days. But that's all."

During the first week, Tucker lost almost 10 pounds. After ten weeks, he was down 41.38 pounds of fat and had reduced the size of his waist by 6.625 inches.

Why Superhydration?

As I stated earlier, superhydration is the name I've attached to drinking 1 gallon of ice-cold water a day. I've applied it since 1985, and all my Gainesville Health & Fitness trainees have used this practice to assist both their fat-loss and muscle-building goals. In fact, with some of my biggest individuals, such as Tucker, I've had them drink up to 1½ gallons a day.

For the record, superhydration:

- Facilitates your liver's ability to metabolize stored fat into energy.
- Forces your body to warm the cold fluid to core body temperature and eliminate it through urine. To warm 1 ounce of 32°F water to 98.6°F (body temperature) requires 1.1 calories of internal heat. Thus, 1 gallon burns 140.8 calories (128 ounces x 1.1 calories) of heat, which is a seldom-practiced way to transfer fat.
- Combats appetite by helping your digestive organs feel full.
- Relieves constipation by softening ingested fiber and keeping food moving through your intestines.
- Hydrates the skin for a smoother, glowing, more youthful complexion.
- Assists the muscle-building process, because your muscles are 72 percent water.

Superhydration warning: Anyone with a kidney disorder, or taking diuretics, should consult with a physician before trying superhydration.

Superhydration Guidelines

How do you drink a gallon of ice-cold water a day? Although such a recommendation may sound difficult, in fact, it only presents a few minor problems—such as how, when, and where. Each of these problems can be solved with some intelligent preparation and careful planning.

How: One tip is to not gulp the water, but sip it. Get yourself one of those 32-ounce plastic bottles, the kind that has a long straw in the top. (I've found that most people can consume water more easily with a straw than trying to gulp it down the standard way from a glass.) Some people prefer a smaller 20-ounce bottle, as opposed to a 32-ounce bottle. There are other sizes, too. The choice is up to you. Just make sure you calculate how many times you'll need to refill the bottle each day to ensure you drink 128 total ounces of water. Also, while you're checking out various bottles, select one that is insulated. The insulation will keep your water colder for a longer time.

When: Try to consume 50 percent before noon and the rest before six p.m. Drinking most of the water earlier in the day may eliminate the need to get out of bed to visit the bathroom during the night. Several of my dieters have commented that getting up in the middle of the night to urinate, then going back to bed, leaves them feeling dehydrated. If that's a feeling you have, it's fine to drink from 4 to 8 ounces of water after late-night urination.

Where: You sip water everywhere you go during the day because you know how to plan ahead. Once again, you need an insulated bottle. But what about refilling the bottle, the ice, and all that hassle of keeping count of the ounces?

The really motivated people invest in a 2-gallon thermos jug. First thing in the morning, they fill the large jug with ice and water. Then they draw off their initial 32 ounces of fluid into their insulated bottle and start sipping. As soon as the bottle is empty, it's refilled from the thermos jug. When they leave home each day, they carry both the thermos jug and the smaller bottle with them. That way, they always have access to their chilled water. When they return home that night, they carefully wash the jug and the bottle so they're ready to use again the next morning.

Some bottle designs are much easier than others. Usually a larger cap, or a cap at both ends, makes the cleaning easier and eliminates the buildup of mildew. Rinsing with water that contains a little diluted bleach can be an effective way to sanitize a bottle. If you have a spare bottle, this allows more time for the first to dry. One tip, if you fall behind, is to speed things up with a hair dryer.

A great way to keep count of how much water you've consumed is to place rubber bands around the middle of the bottle, with each rubber band representing a number of ounces. Each time you finish that many ounces, take off a rubber band and put it in your pocket. For example, if you have a 32-ounce water bottle, you'll need four rubber bands (four 32-ounce bottles equal 1 gallon), or remove and then add back two rubber bands.

Additives: There is a difference between plain water and beverages that contain mostly water. Those mostly water liquids—such as soft drinks, coffee, tea, beer, and fruit juices—also contain sugar, flavors, caffeine, and alcohol. Sugar and alcohol add calories. Caffeine—found in coffee, tea, and many soft drinks—stimulates the adrenal glands and acts as a diuretic. Rather than superhydrate the system, caffeine-containing beverages actually dehydrate the body. You should keep your consumption of such beverages to a minimum.

The only flavoring I recommend for water is a twist of lemon or lime, and most people who initially like adding lemon or lime eventually get to the point where they prefer their water plain.

Tap water or bottled water: The decision to consume bottled water or tap is usually one of preference. In general, the United States has one of the safest water supplies in the world. Chances are high that your community's tap water or the water from your well is fine for drinking. The main concern is the presence of chlorine in city water. Chlorine, as pool owners know, evaporates, so if you fill a jug with tap water and leave it out on the counter for 6–8 hours before pouring it into your container, the chlorine will have evaporated.

Research shows that bottled water is not always higher-quality water than tap water. In fact, many bottled waters are simply city water in a plastic bottle. Some questions have been raised about the plastic used for the bottles, especially during the summer. Different companies use different plastic for their bottles. Some use glass, although this tends to be more costly and cumbersome, because of its extra weight and fragility. There has also been a trend toward stainless-steel bottles.

If you dislike the taste of your tap water, drink your favorite bottled water. Just be sure to check the label carefully and avoid any water with additives. If you have no problems with your city's water supply or the water from your well, then save some money and drink that.

Helpful Notes from Ted Tucker

- The water drinking was difficult at first, with so many bathroom breaks, but that also got me standing and moving, which was better for me than long hours of just sitting. Plus, with all that internal flow, my entire system felt cleaner. That was such a great feeling. I now love the taste of water.
- Interestingly, I've tracked my drinking and restroom visits. On a typical day, spread over 13 hours, my water intake totals an average of 140 ounces. That's a little over 1 gallon. Almost 1.1 gallons of water results in fifteen restroom visits. That seems like a lot of toilet time, which it is. But it's worth it, especially since every ounce of urine puts me closer to my leanest, strongest, healthiest body.
- It took me almost a week to get my system adapted to the chilled water. At first my bladder seemed to be extra sensitive, and I urinated twenty-two times a day. But after the first week, my bladder adjusted and I could hold it longer, and I settled in at fifteen times daily.
- Superhydration has been a wonderful addition to my life. I use it to burn calories, curb hunger, nourish my muscles, hydrate my skin, flush my system, and keep me active. It will do the same for you. Get involved now and enjoy the benefits.

The Circle of Water

The earth's water circle, cycle, or rotation describes how water evaporates from the surface of the earth, rises into the atmosphere, cools and condenses in clouds, and falls again as precipitation. The precipitation collects in lakes and rivers, and on soil and rocks, and much of it flows back into the oceans.

Water on earth involves a marvel of equilibrium. The distance between the sun and the earth keeps ground temperatures almost perfect for allowing water to remain in a gaseous or solid state, thus preventing large-scale flooding. Without the atmospheric blanket that shields and safeguards the earth, the water cycle would not exist, and life as we know it would never have evolved.

The most extraordinary fact is that the water that is so present and necessary in our lives, the water that permeates and superhydrates each one of our cells—this same water was here in the earth's early stages more than four billion years ago.

In its three stages . . . gas, liquid, and solid . . . the circle of water endures without end.

Think about it—with superhydration, you are now more actively involved than ever in the circle of water.

Shall we drink to it?

18

BROWN FAT METABOLISM

MAKING YOUR FAT CELLS WORK FOR YOU

THE MOST COMMON fat on your body, as discussed in chapter 4, is white fat, which is stored primarily around your belly, torso, hips, and upper thighs. White fat is where your body stores fuel for the long term and can be mobilized for energy. It has a limited blood supply, making it white in color.

Another type of fat in the body is brown fat, which is light brown in color due to its rich blood supply and numerous pigmented mitochondria. Brown fat is most commonly found in babies, around the neck, collarbones, and spine. Babies lack the ability to shiver, so their bodies use brown fat to keep warm in times of unexpected temperature drops. Until recently, it was thought that this brown fat disappeared after early infancy. However, an important study reported in the *New England Journal of Medicine* in 2009 concluded that many, perhaps all, adults still have stores of brown fat. More recently, in 2014, a study published in *Cell Metabolism* reported that it was possible—under the right conditions—for adults to turn some white fat cells into brown fat cells.

How do you get your dormant brown fat cells to reemerge and reignite? The answer is adaptive thermodynamics. On the following pages, I've described various ways you can involve adaptive thermodynamics in your weight loss program.

Expose Your Skin to Cold Temperatures

Cold temperatures send a signal to the brain that stimulates brown fat activity in two ways: by acting on your vascular system directly to increase blood flow to your brown fat stores, and by sending nerve impulses to brown fat cells that provide an additional boost in cellular actions.

How cold do you have to be? A Japanese research team found that sitting in a 59°F room for two hours wearing summer clothing will stimulate brown fat to burn an extra 100 to 250 calories. The researchers also found that half the test subjects under age thirty-eight showed signs of brown fat activation in a 66°F setting. Results were less impressive for people older than thirty-eight.

Activate Brown Fat with Cold Feet

In one study, Swedish researchers scanned five subjects after they'd spent two hours at temperatures ranging between 63°F and 66°F. During the scan itself, the subjects cooled their body temperatures even further by repeatedly placing one foot in ice water for 5 minutes at a time, followed by 5 minutes out of the water, then doing the same with the other foot.

The scientists reported that not only did all the subjects have detectable brown fat deposits, but that the added foot exposure to the ice water boosted their brown fat activity fifteenfold.

Do Your Workouts in Cool Temperatures

Boost the number of calories you burn during exercise by stimulating your brown fat stores during your workouts. How? Exercise in a setting kept at 64°F or lower. Even better: Make sure your skin is uncovered, because the evaporation of sweat as you exercise adds to the cooling effect.

What you *don't* want to do: Increase your perspiration by turning up the heat when you exercise. The hotter environment will actually shut down brown fat activity.

Stimulate Your Body's Melatonin Production

The hormone melatonin helps regulate our sleep-wake cycles. Research published in the *Journal of Pineal Research* reported that in rats, melatonin increases the presence of "beige" fat, which is similar to brown fat in its calorie-burning abilities.

Experts say that rather than taking a melatonin supplement, it's best to stimulate your body's natural production of melatonin by avoiding nighttime exposure to light from computers and other screens, getting 20 minutes of sunlight exposure most days, and loading up on melatonin-rich foods such as almonds, peanuts, tomatoes, and broccoli.

Improve Your Blood Sugar Metabolism with More Brown Fat

Brown fat may have unique diabetes-fighting properties. People with lower glucose levels tend to have more brown fat than those with higher levels, which indicates that it may play a role in blood sugar.

For example, one group of investigators found that a certain protein in brown fat appears to enhance the metabolism of white fat. When they studied a strain of experimental mice who were lacking this protein, they found that the mice expended less energy, gained weight, and developed diabetes.

In another study, a research team transplanted a small amount of brown fat into the abdomens of a group of mice. After eight weeks, the mice given the transplants were not only leaner than a placebo group, but also processed glucose better and had reduced insulin resistance.

Increase Your Metabolic Set Point with More Brown Fat

Set point is the body weight at which the brain automatically begins to slow metabolic rate, making it more difficult to remove additional flab. By stoking metabolic activity, brown fat could help combat the metabolic slowdown that occurs when people start dropping significant fat. If someone is able to burn an extra 200 or 300 calories a day through their brown fat, that is enough to shed a pound of body fat in just a couple of weeks.

As Americans get older, they typically add 10 pounds of fat per decade. The calorie-burning advance from brown fat could be enough to combat or reverse this weight gain and help older individuals maintain the fat percentage they had as young adults.

Consider a Low-Fat, High-Carbohydrate Eating Plan

Radiologists want to decrease brown fat activity when doing scans of cancer patients, because the heat generated by brown fat makes it harder to see tumor-related activity. As a consequence, they recommend that patients eat high-fat, low-carbohydrate diets before scans, since such diets reduce brown fat activation. This suggests that a low-fat, high-carbohydrate diet—such as the one I recommend in this book, will enhance brown fat activity.

Eat More Apples, Including the Peel

New research shows that ursolic acid—a substance that occurs in high concentrations in apple skins—increases brown fat and muscle mass, while at the same time reducing fat and improving glucose tolerance. If you don't like apples, other foods that contain ursolic acid include cranberries, blueberries, plums, and prunes.

Take Charge of Your Thermostat

Turning the thermostat down in your bedroom to 66°F significantly increases your nightly metabolism and caloric burn. Scientists at the National Institutes of Health Clinical Center examined how long-term exposure to moderately cold temperatures affected fat cells in five healthy male volunteers. The volunteers spent four consecutive months sleeping in temperature-controlled rooms. Only a single sheet was available as a cover for each participant. During the day, the participants were allowed to perform their activities as normal.

The following protocol was used: Researchers kept the overnight temperature at 75°F for the first month, followed by 66°F for the second month, 75°F for the third month, and 81°F for the fourth. The collected data showed that the men doubled their brown fat volume and improved insulin sensitivity after sleeping in the 66°F room for a month. Sleeping in the higher-temperature environments had no effect on their brown fat and even suppressed it.

I've found that most of my research subjects can adapt, within several weeks, to sleeping in a cooler bedroom. In the winter, you can keep the heat low, lighten your covers, shun electric blankets, and even practice keeping one leg uncovered.

IN no time, you'll get the hang of applying adaptive thermodynamics on your inner and outer body. And your emerging brown fat will give your metabolism a significant boost.

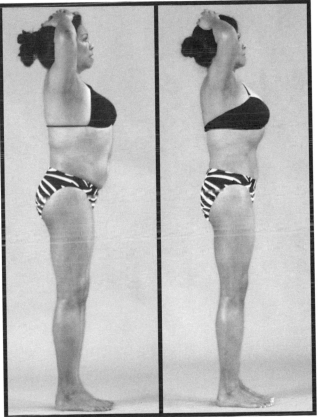

157.7 pounds   140.75 pounds

MARLENE HILL, age 59, height 5'6"
AFTER 6 WEEKS
20.12 pounds of fat loss
4 inches off waist
3.17 pounds of muscle gain

19

THE COLD PLUNGE

YOUR SKIN, CONDUCTION, AND ALTERNATIVES

THE COLD PLUNGE at Gainesville Health & Fitness is a 4-foot-deep, 6-by-8-foot pool filled with 52°F water. Near the bottom of the pool are regulators to keep the water at the desired temperature. As many as four people can get into the cold plunge at the same time.

"I Could Hardly Believe the Transformation"

"The cold plunge literally sucked the fat right out of my body," Javier Woody said. "I lost twenty pounds in the first three weeks. I could hardly believe the transformation."

When I met, measured, and photographed Woody on October 19, 2017, he was twenty-one years of age, stood 5 feet 10 inches tall, and weighed 233.6 pounds. His body fat percentage was 33.6 and his waist measured 45.625 inches. I figured he could lose 20 pounds of fat in six weeks, not three, but I also didn't expect him to hit the cold plunge five times a week for three consecutive weeks.

How was Woody able to get the fat out of his body so fast?

Some of the answer had to do with the Killing Fat program's lower-calorie diet and negative-accentuated exercise. But a surprising part of the answer is that he forced the heat out through his skin. Woody's 5-feet-10-inch body, with a protruding waist, had a large surface area. More surface area means a larger rug could be made from your hide. A larger rug means the possibility of more effective conduction.

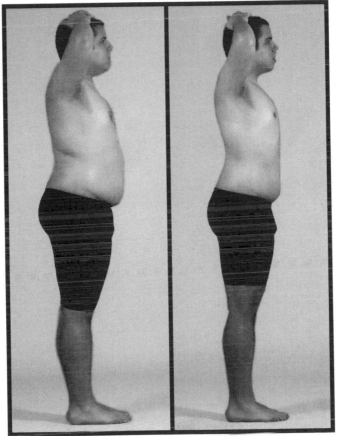

233.6 pounds   195.4 pounds

JAVIER WOODY, age 21, height 5'10"

AFTER 8 WEEKS

43.32 pounds of fat loss

7.125 inches off waist

5.12 pounds of muscle gain

Conduction

Conduction in this context is the transfer of heat calories from the skin into the colder water. When Woody eased into the cold water, his core body temperature of 98.6°F, in an attempt to keep his body warm in the 52°F water, produced significant heat calories. Thus, conduction occurred from his skin to the water. The more skin available to the cold water, the better the conduction and transfer of heat.

My belief is that Woody ignited 50 calories per minute in the cold plunge. In 10 minutes, that's equal to 500 calories of heat, or 500 calories of fat.

Water is a much better conductor than air, so you can get rid of more calories in cold water than cold air. Drinking chilled water, which I discussed in chapter 17, is another way to take advantage of conduction. To be almost shivering is another example of conduction, and also stimulates your adrenal glands to produce noradrenaline—which, in turn, causes your body to burn more calories. Also, the above practices stimulate your brown fat cells to jump into action.

Besides conduction, your body transfers heat through your skin in several other ways.

Convection and Evaporation

Convection is a process in which heat is transferred by the movement of gases or liquids (like air or water). That's why wind makes you feel cooler when you are walking, cycling, or running outdoors. Or why an overhead fan in an exercise room can benefit the heat-loss process.

While you may not be aware of it, your skin perspires constantly, even when you're not exercising. This unnoticeable perspiration is eliminated by evaporation. At ordinary room temperatures, the moisture vaporized from your skin plus that expelled from your lungs when you exhale accounts for substantial calories lost from your body at rest.

Radiation

Another way heat is transferred through the skin is radiation. Significant calories are eliminated through your skin each day as radiant heat. Radiation is one reason why a tall person has an easier time dropping fat than a shorter person of the same weight. Taller people, compared to shorter ones, have more skin surface area available to the environment and thus can radiate more heat.

Few people realize that the skin is the body's largest organ. An average woman's skin, if it were laid out flat, would cover approximately 20 square feet. An average man's skin would cover more like 23.4 square feet.

Remember, the more skin surface area you have, the better your body is able to transfer your unwanted fat through radiation, evaporation, convection, and conduction.

BACK TO THE COLD PLUNGE: HOW TO GET THE BEST RESULTS

If you want to get the best fat-loss results from using a cold plunge, here are the important points to follow:

- Wear a tight-fitting bathing suit. Billowing pant legs are bothersome.
- Check the temperature gauge; it should read between 52°F and 54°F.

- Don't assume that colder is better. Spending time in water colder than 52°F can be dangerous. On the other hand, 60°F to 75°F water can still be beneficial.
- Have a clock with a second hand nearby so you can note the time you spend in the water. Ten minutes is your target goal.
- Do not wear rubber boots or rubber gloves. Your feet and hands emit a large amount of heat, so take advantage of this.
- Ease into the water by walking down the stairs. Your midsection is usually a difficult area to submerge. If so, take 30 seconds to inch your way down.
- Get your hands and arms into the water.
- Try to breathe normally.
- Submerge your chest and shoulders and think nice thoughts. Moving your feet and hands may be helpful.
- Discussing the topics of the day with another cold plunger is often helpful.
- Keep breathing as normally as possible.
- Check the clock. After 3 or 4 minutes, the process gets somewhat easier.
- Some people choose to work up to 10 minutes over the course of a week, by going from 6 to 7 to 8 to 9 and finally to 10 minutes.
- Exit the pool at the 10-minute mark. Do not exceed 10 minutes.
- Sit near the pool for several minutes and regain your senses.
- Stand, walk back to the dressing room, and take a warm shower.
- Enjoy your ride home.

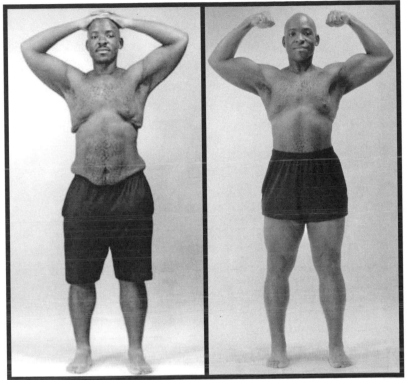

208.5 pounds   194.75 pounds

CLIFTON POWELL, age 26, height 5'10"
AFTER 6 WEEKS
24.28 pounds of fat loss
5 inches off waist
10.53 pounds of muscle gain

Be Alert: Avoid the Cold Plunge
Immediately After Strength Training

I've made this mistake, and some of my trainees have, too. It's a good idea to wait for an hour after a negative-accentuated strength-training session before going into the cold plunge. Here's why:

My 30–10–30, negative-accentuated form of strength training generates a lot of muscular inflammation, which is a good thing. Your body needs most of this inflammation to maximize growth. Too much, however, causes extreme soreness in your body.

The cold plunge causes an anti-inflammatory response, which you want to blunt some of the soreness, but not so much that it removes some of the immediate *inflammatory* action from your negative-accentuated workout. Research shows that waiting for an hour after your strength training is an appropriate time for both processes to be utilized effectively.

Cold Plunge Alternatives

If you don't have access to a cold plunge, here are a couple of alternatives to try. Again, wait for an hour after a strength-training session before trying either method.

A COLD SHOWER:
- Use hot water for 1 to 2 minutes over your entire body.
- Step out of the hot water and apply shampoo to your hair. Lather up.
- Switch the water to pure cold and rinse your head and face alone.
- Rotate and back quickly into the cold water. Focus the spray on your lower neck and upper back.
- Maintain this position for 1 to 3 minutes. As you acclimatize, soap the rest of your body.
- Turn around and rinse normally.
- Exit the shower and towel yourself dry.

An ice pack for your neck: Try placing a U-shaped ice pack around the back of your neck and upper trapezius for approximately 30 minutes in the evening three times per week. Several of my trainees in Orlando tried this technique and were reasonably pleased with the results.

HANGING SKIN AND ADDED MUSCLE: WHAT WORKED FOR ONE MAN

Clifton Powell was a hardworking trainee at Gainesville Health & Fitness who had an issue with hanging skin. Powell had lost 56 pounds during the preceding year on a lower-calorie diet of his own design. During that time, he did no strength training. His "before" photo on page 235 revealed several inches of hanging skin over the sides of his chest and waist.

During the Killing Fat program, Powell trained intensely and followed the eating and water-drinking schedule consistently for six weeks. He also used the cold plunge. His hanging skin shrank significantly. His muscularity also improved dramatically, as he built 10.53 pounds of muscle and added 0.5 inch to each upper arm.

Surgery is the only way to remove the skin permanently, but that doesn't mean it's right for everyone. It involves general anesthesia, suturing, significant recovery time, and scarring. It's also costly, and most patients have to pay out of pocket, as insurance rarely covers cosmetic surgery.

My safest advice for hanging skin is to get the fat off, continue to stay hydrated, use the cold plunge, dress appropriately, and be patient. And pay attention to Clifton Powell's best direction: "Build your muscles . . . and keep building them."

SLEEP BLITZING AND BOMBING

GETTING 8½ TO 10 HOURS A NIGHT

I'**VE TOLD THE** following story to some of my Killing Fat groups, and it's worth sharing here.

A Soldier's Experience

"This heavy negative-accentuated exercise makes my body hungry for more sleep," Shane Poole said. "More sleep immediately after the workout, and more sleep for at least three consecutive nights."

That was unexpected, coming from a big, strong, young man who from 2006 through 2009 thrived on five hours of sleep a night in Iraq, where he was a unit weapons sergeant in the U.S. Army.

Poole—now a college student in Gainesville—continued: "Being around explosives constantly in Iraq did not prepare me for the deep stimulation and the more-sleep requirement that was necessary for the muscular growth that I wanted."

When I announced in March 2012 that I was organizing a group of fifteen men who wanted to build significant muscle (and did not

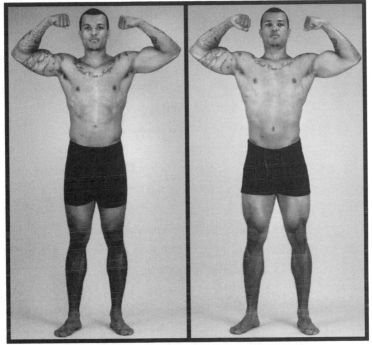

204.5 pounds   224 pounds

SHANE POOLE, age 28, height 6'3"

AFTER 6 WEEKS

(on muscle building program only)

19.5 pounds of muscle gain

1.5 inches added on arms

3.75 inches added on thighs

need to lose fat), Poole signed up first. The plan was for me to train each man with negative-accentuated techniques once a week for six consecutive weeks. Poole had heard me talking about rapid-rate muscular growth, and he told me he was going to work harder than anyone else.

He didn't disappoint.

Before his first workout, Poole stood 6 feet 3 inches tall, had 6.6 percent body fat, and weighed 204.5 pounds. After his sixth workout, with no change in his body fat, Poole weighed 224 pounds. That was a gain of 19.5 pounds of solid muscle in six weeks.

"I Needed 10 Hours"

"I realized after my first workout," Poole remembered, "as I was lying on the cool dressing room floor, that I couldn't keep my eyes open. Within thirty seconds, I was out—not unconscious—but stone-cold asleep. I was out on that hard tile floor for an hour . . . an entire hour.

"I finally got up, spent five minutes in the cold plunge, showered, drove home, ate supper. I turned the air conditioner down as low as it would go and went to bed . . . and slept for another nine hours.

"And I continued to sleep for a good nine hours each of the next three nights . . . plus an hour nap every afternoon. I couldn't believe it. Most mornings, I'd roll out of bed and look in the mirror and think, 'OMG, I'm bigger.' And I was larger and stronger."

Poole did not initially know, but soon appreciated, that the vast majority of muscular growth occurs during sleep. Negative exercise forced him to sleep deeper and longer. And turning down the thermostat enhanced his sleep. Applying bodybuilding terminology, he was blitzing and bombing his muscle and fat with precision productivity.

Precision Productivity

Most people who are trying to fight fat need to grasp that at least 50 percent of their daily fat loss occurs while they are sleeping. This is especially true if you are on a 1,500-calorie-a-day eating plan combined with a rigorous exercise routine.

In addition to the diet and exercise plan, to make the entire Killing Fat program really work, I want you to focus on three important practices:

1. Get at least 8½ hours of sleep a night . . . 10 hours is even better.
2. Be less active during the day and night.
3. Try to take a 30-minute afternoon nap.

What makes those three practices so important—besides the fact that they worked for Shane Poole and most of the other people in the Killing Fat program in Gainesville—is that they are based on science.

Let's closely examine this research.

Sleep: A Powerful Fat-Loss Tool

In a study published in the *Annals of Internal Medicine* in 2010, titled "Insufficient Sleep Undermines Dietary Efforts to Reduce Adiposity," Dr. Arlet Nedeltcheva and his colleagues compared two groups of overfat people who were each fed 1,450 calories per day for fourteen days. One group logged 8½ hours of sleep per night, and the other clocked 5½ hours per night (which the authors noted is the "norm" for most adults today). After two weeks, the people who slept longer had lost significantly more fat than the group who slept less.

Most dieters do not do strength training at the same time they are eating less and end up losing both fat and muscle—as did both the group getting 8½ hours of sleep and the group getting 5½ hours. But get this: The sleep-deprived group dropped 60 percent more muscle than the group who slept more. Those three hours of missing sleep caused a shift in metabolism that made the body want to preserve fat at the expense of muscle.

That was not all. When the researchers compared circulating blood levels of appetite-regulating hormones in the two groups, they found that those who slept for three fewer hours produced more of the appetite-stimulating hormone ghrelin. In other words, they woke up hungrier than the group who slept more.

Many people assume their bodies burn more calories when they are awake longer, but that is not the case. The metabolic rate is down-regulated with less sleep. In other words, when you sleep less, your body starts to burn calories at a slower rate to preserve energy.

Here's another significant finding: In the same study, participants burned on average *400 more calories by sleeping for three more hours.* That's an additional 2,800 calories in one week, or 5,600 calories in two weeks—which is very significant.

With less sleep, the body seeks to meet the increased metabolic needs of longer waking hours by shifting into a lower gear that burns more muscle and less fat. That is certainly not the type of fat-loss program you want to be involved with.

To sum this up, if you want to preserve muscle, burn fat, and wake up less hungry when you are dieting, sleep for at least 8½ hours a night.

Inactivity: A Powerful Muscle-Building Tool

For more than forty years, Arthur Jones, the man who invented Nautilus strength-training machines, explored the concept of *If a muscle is stimulated to grow, when does it actually grow?* He could never boil it down to an exact time, but he did establish the following:

- Muscular growth, once it is stimulated, requires inactivity. It will not grow if you are overly involved in various sports or fitness activities on non-training days. To make sure you get stronger, firmer muscles from exercise, you must rest more.
- More than 90 percent of muscular growth occurs during sleep, and probably during a deep-sleep period of only 5 to 10 minutes.
- If in doubt about how much rest and sleep to get, error on the side of too much rather than too little.

During the research for my Body Fat Breakthrough program at Gainesville Health & Fitness, I observed some revealing behaviors among participants in the intense negative-accentuated exercise program.

This negative-accentuated training made a deeper inroad into a participant's starting level of strength, perhaps 40 to 50 percent deeper than with normal training. Such deeper inroads triggered the production of at least six hormones: growth hormone, insulin-like growth factor, mechano-growth factor, interleukin-6, interleukin-15, and insulin. The effects of these hormones on the human body were fatigue, rest, and deep sleep—and they all occurred *quickly*. Remember Shane Poole's story? Poole was not the only guy who experienced the cool floor in the dressing room.

Such observations lead to the next research finding.

Naps Can Help Your Results

In addition to getting 8½ hours of sleep each night, I'm now asking you to take an afternoon nap, right? Yes, that's correct. Here's why.

In 2005, Cheri Mah, MS, a researcher at the Stanford Sleep Disorders Clinic, asked members of Stanford's varsity basketball team to try to sleep more. Every one of them did and in doing so improved their performance in sprinting, free-throw shooting, and three point shooting.

Such findings eventually caught the attention of a number of NBA players, such as Steve Nash, Kobe Bryant, and Lebron James—all of whom slept more, liked it, and performed better. "Many athletes have optimized physical training and recovery," Mah said. "There really hasn't been the same emphasis on optimizing sleep and recovery."

The Stanford players and the interested NBA athletes were all encouraged to nap every day. Daily naps were like a magic pill to them. Even a brief nap can help the body release crucial growth hormones—which stimulate the healing of muscle and bone.

Enter Dr. Charles Czeisler, a professor at Harvard Medical School and today's go-to expert for professional sports teams from every major league. He noted that sleep deprivation could lead to high blood pressure, depression, and weight gain, as well as poor athletic performance. What many athletes don't recognize is that it's the sleep after a game, or even after an intense workout, that's most important.

Plus, Czeisler said, a 30-minute midafternoon nap could do wonders for recovery. And that's precisely 30 minutes—no less and no more.

In my opinion, a midafternoon nap not only helps muscle recovery, but also contributes to fat loss. I've seen it happen many times with my own eyes.

Effective Napping Strategies

If you've never napped, it may take a little effort. Here are four guidelines:

Time it right: Try to nap between two and four p.m., the time your circadian cycle dips. Napping later in the day may make it more difficult to fall asleep at night.

Set an alarm: Napping for longer than 30 minutes may leave you groggy and disrupt your nighttime sleep.

Nap in bed: A cool, dark room will help you rest better.

Don't hit the snooze button: When the alarm goes off, get right up. Walk around, splash water on your face, do a few jumping jacks—anything to wake you up and make you active again.

THE LATEST RESEARCH ON SLEEP

For a better understanding of sleep, let's examine some of the latest facts about it.

- We sleep less as we age. An infant sleeps 14 hours a day; a healthy teenager averages 9½ hours; and people over seventy-five years old manage only 6 hours.

- We naturally feel tired at two different times of the day: about two a.m. and two p.m.
- According to the *International Classifications of Sleep Disorders*, shift workers are at increased risk for a variety of chronic illnesses, such as cardiovascular, and gastrointestinal diseases.
- We have lost our natural rhythms. The essential one, with some variation during the year because of longer or shorter days, is the circadian rhythm. This is basically the 24-hour, or daily, rhythm.
- Before the era of electricity, it wasn't difficult to stay synchronized with the circadian rhythm, because we couldn't see to plow the fields or bring in the harvest except between dawn and dusk. Our hormonal cycles have stayed in this original rhythm rather than adapting to the electric light revolution of the past century; from an evolutionary perspective, adaptation in such a short time is unlikely.
- The key nighttime hormone is melatonin, and it's easily disrupted by exposure to light, even artificial light.
- Snoring is the primary cause of sleep disruption for approximately 90 million American adults.
- According to the results of the National Sleep Foundation's Sleep in America poll, 36 percent of Americans drive drowsy or fall asleep while driving.
- People who don't get enough sleep are more likely to have bigger appetites due to the fact that their levels of leptin, an appetite-regulating hormone, fall, promoting appetite increase.
- The latest figures from the National Sleep Foundation show that the average adult in the United States gets 6 hours 57 minutes sleep per night during the workweek and 7 hours 31 minutes sleep per night during weekends.

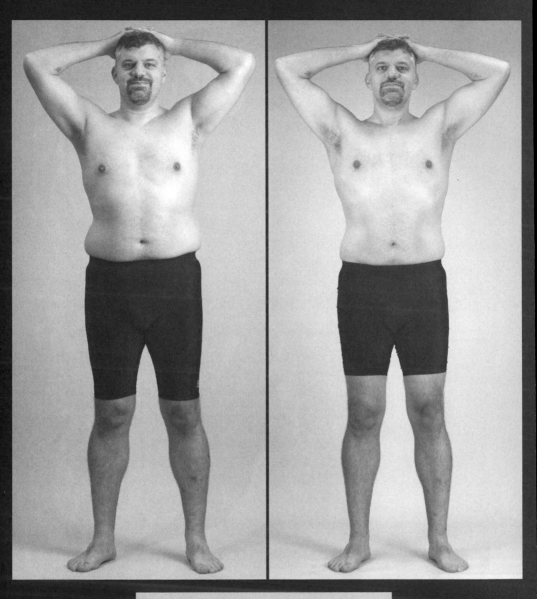

251 pounds   **223** pounds

WAYNE PARE, age 39, height 6'
AFTER 12 WEEKS
34.29 pounds of fat loss
8.375 inches off waist
6.29 pounds of muscle gain

Part V

YOUR *KILLING FAT BODY* FOR LIFE

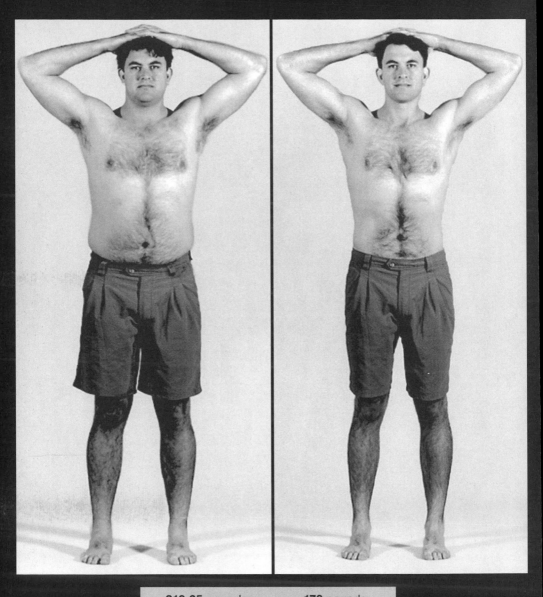

219.25 pounds   **170** pounds

JEFF ARNOLD, age 27, height 6'1"

AFTER 12 WEEKS

54.25 pounds of fat loss

8.25 inches off waist

5 pounds of muscle gain

21

"TELL ME WHY?"

YOUR QUESTIONS ANSWERED

Q: *Is it okay if I occasionally shift the lunch selections to dinner and the dinner selections to lunch?*

A: Yes, this is fine, as long as it is only done occasionally. You must be careful that you do not get into the habit of shifting things around too often. This leads to a lackadaisical attitude and soon your entire diet becomes very unstructured.

Q: *What about skipping breakfast and making up the calories at another meal? Is this okay?*

A: No. Most dieters who skip breakfast have the tendency to snack later or to overeat at their next meal. They actually end up by consuming more calories for the day.

Get into the habit of eating breakfast, and do not skip meals.

Q: *During the first couple of weeks on the Killing Fat diet, I got very hungry. Any tips on how to fight such hunger?*

A: You're not experiencing true hunger. True hunger occurs from severe food deprivation. You'd have to be in a starving situation for many weeks or months to reach such a state. What you're suffering from is false hunger. Your appetite is simply trying to get your attention. Remember in part I when I described the appetite-controlling mechanism in your brain (see page 43)?

There are several guides you can use to keep your appetite in check. First, don't go longer than three hours between your small meals. Carbohydrate-rich foods trigger the right signals to your brain. Second, get up and move around. Being active raises your internal temperature, which also helps.

Q: *I'm confused. All my training buddies, when they want to lose fat, avoid eating carbohydrates. Please help me understand why eating carbohydrates is essential in fat loss.*

A: I appreciate where you are coming from, and I know how tough it is to go against what many of your friends believe and practice. Normally, a complete discussion of the importance of carbohydrates in a college nutrition textbook would take twenty pages or more. I'm going to condense it to five paragraphs and hope that you get the essence of why carbs are key. Let's begin by examining glucose.

Glucose: Glucose is the basic carbohydrate unit used for energy by each of your body's cells. The cells of your brain and nervous system depend almost exclusively on glucose, and your red blood cells use glucose alone. Only dietary carbohydrates release glucose, and that's why carbs are classified as an essential nutrient. For vigorous health, you need plenty of them each day to power your body and brain.

Lack of carbohydrates: Although you can eat too many carbohydrates and the extra glucose can be converted to body fat, body fat cannot be converted to glucose to feed your brain adequately. When your body faces a severe carbohydrate deficit, it has two problems: Having no glucose, it has to make glucose from proteins, which, because of proteins' critical functions, it does not like to do, even in emergencies. When it is forced to do so, it pulls proteins from your organs and muscles—which makes no sense, especially if you are interested in fitness and health. Carbohydrates should be available to prevent your body from stealing proteins from your muscles for energy. This is called the protein-sparing action of carbohydrates. Remember, protein builds muscle, and muscle burns a lot of calories. If your body cannibalizes its muscle to make glucose to feed your brain, you compromise one of your body's prime natural calorie burners. You need adequate carbohydrates every day. Don't starve yourself of carbs, but do choose them wisely.

Ketone bodies: The second problem with a lack of dietary carbohydrates is a precarious shift in your body's energy metabolism. Instead of following the carbohydrate-energy pathway, fats are forced to fragment and combine with each other—which causes an accumulation of normally scarce acidic products called ketone bodies. Ketone bodies can accumulate in the blood to disturb the body's normal acid-base balance, which then may promote deficiencies of vitamins and minerals, elevate blood cholesterol, and yield little energy. As a result, most low-carbohydrate dieters soon feel lethargic and have poor motivation.

Minimum recommendation for carbohydrates: To provide glucose, preserve proteins (and muscle mass), and avoid ketone bodies, you need to consume adequate carbohydrates each day. According to the National Institutes of Health's Dietary Reference Intakes (DRI) for healthy adults in the United States, the minimum amount of dietary carbohydrates is 130 grams—which equals 520 calories of carbohydrate-rich foods each day. The Killing Fat menus furnish an average of 650 calories or more each day of carbohydrate-rich foods—such as fruits, vegetables, and whole grains.

In summary, for effective fat loss and efficient belly blasting, a healthy man or woman needs at least 130 grams of carbohydrates a day to supply glucose for brain alertness, initiate protein-sparing action, prevent ketone bodies, and provide energy for training and daily activities. The Killing Fat diet contains the right amount of carbohydrates, combined with proteins, fats, and water, to make your journey successful.

Q: *Are you saying all of the popular low-carbohydrate diets do not work?*

A: What I'm saying is these diets, without adequate carbohydrates, do not work competently to help you lose fat. If you are only interested in losing weight, not fat, then eliminating carbohydrates will result in a loss of water from your body. Remember, carbohydrates are *hydrated carbons*. Each ounce of glucose carries 3 ounces of water. Go on a low-carbohydrate diet for a week and you may lose 5 or 6 pounds of water weight. The water, however, will not drain from your fat. It will come from your organs and muscles. But the typical low-carbohydrate dieter won't recognize that detail.

Since most people rarely endure strict low-carbohydrate dieting on their own for longer than two weeks, the initial scale drop from the loss of water provides them with a false sense of achievement. Many then believe that if they had continued the diet for longer, they would have reached their goal. Thus, the low-carbohydrate eating practices appear to work when in fact they don't, and these beliefs continue to be reinforced.

Remember, low-carbohydrate diets are based on opinions, not laws.

As I discussed in part I, your goal should be to lose fat and build your underlying muscles. In fact, building muscle at the same time that you are losing weight ensures that your weight loss comes from your fat cells.

That's one of the primary reasons a carbohydrate-rich eating plan is important in the Killing Fat program.

Eating plans that advise people to avoid carbohydrates supplied by fruits, vegetables, and breads should be ignored. Enjoying tasty carbohydrates within your daily calorie limit is a part of the Killing Fat diet. As you progress through the complete program—and see and feel significant results—you'll appreciate carbohydrates more and more.

Q: *I was impressed by your before-and-after photos of Joe Walker* [see page 56]. *You noted that he was on a muscle-building-only program. Can you describe this program?*

A: Walker was a bodybuilder, who had well-above-average genetics for developing large muscles. In the summer of 2012, I put Walker and fourteen other guys through a negative-accentuated program for six weeks. The majority of the men were trained only once a week, on exercises similar to the routines described in chapter 14. Where the program differed from the Killing Fat plan was that the men had no calorie restrictions. They were encouraged to eat from 3,000 to 3,600 calories a day and superhydrate their systems daily with 1 gallon of water.

The two guys who did the best were Walker and Shane Poole (who was featured in chapter 20).

Q: *You talk about measuring body fat using a Lange skinfold caliper in chapter 10. Exactly how do you determine body fat percentage, and how does this eventually indicate a person's muscle gain?*

A: When I was director of research at Nautilus, I learned the correct technique for applying the Lange skinfold caliper to determine body fat percentages for both men and women. It takes skill and experience in getting accurate and reliable results from this tool. The caliper measures a double fold of skin and attached fat in the favorite storage areas. I use the three site method and formula developed by Jackson and Pollock to determine body fat percentage.

For men, I measure in millimeters the right-side chest, right-side navel, and right-side mid-thigh, then total the three numbers. For women, I measure the right-arm triceps, right-side hip, and right-side mid-thigh, then total the three numbers. The appropriate chart, which depends on gender and age, is then applied to determine body fat percentage.

Once I have a person's body fat percentage, I multiply that number times their body weight in pounds—which gives me their total pounds of body fat. That's an important number: pounds of body fat.

Okay, let's fast-forward and say that person has progressed through the Killing Fat program for six weeks. I retake measurements at the same three sites, using the same caliper, total the three, and determine his new body fat percentage. Take that percentage and multiply it by his new body weight in pounds, and I have his new total pounds of body fat.

What I want to do now is compare the *before* and *after* pounds of body fat. The after number should be smaller than the before number. Then I compare the fat pounds lost to the body weight pounds lost, in which the weight loss should be smaller than the fat loss.

For example, let's say a twenty-five-year-old man has lost 26.5 pounds of body weight over the six-week program. His body fat percentage in the chart reveals he's dropped 34 pounds of fat. He's lost more fat than weight, which is desirable. I subtract his body weight pounds lost from his body fat pounds lost, and the number is 7.5 pounds.

That 7.5-pound difference is an indication that my twenty-five-year-old trainee has gained that much muscle. Yes, it's an indirect measurement, but when you then take that number and co-relate it with his body measurements, before-and-after photographs, and strength-training records, you can judge the accuracy of the skinfold determinations. With my experience in working with thousands of subjects, I know how to double check, compare, and make minor adjustments, if necessary. I also know from experience that 7.5 pounds of muscle gain is reasonable for a young man who has worked hard.

Q: *What's an ideal body fat percentage for a young man?*

A: According to the Jackson and Pollock formula and charts, ideal body fat percentage increases gradually with age. The American Council on Exercise considers the following range ideal for a young man: 6 to 12 percent. I encourage my young men to reach 10 percent, or sometimes lower. At age fifty, a man's ideal range would be 16 to 18 percent. A young woman's ideal would be 16 to 20 percent, and those numbers would increase to 24 to 26 percent at age fifty.

Of course, there is some individual variation depending on genetics, height, race, and geographical factors.

Q: *It seems like you should have different water-drinking recommendations for a man weighing 300 pounds and a woman weighing 150 pounds, yet they are both the same. Shouldn't you revise your recommendations?*

A: In 1996, for several fat-loss groups, I tried the following formula: 1 ounce of water for every 2 pounds of body weight. If you were 300 pounds (man or woman), you would begin with 150 ounces a day. On the other hand, if you were a 150-pound individual, you would start with 75 ounces. Every two weeks, you would recalculate the ounces per day for the next two weeks based on your lower body weight.

This recommendation worked fine in dealing with individuals, and in small groups of five people or fewer. But in large groups of twenty to thirty individuals (both men and women), there tended to be some confusion. And from my point of view, looking at the overall fat-loss results between the groups that used the formula versus the ones that drank 1 gallon per day, there were no significant differences. They all had approximately the same results.

In the Killing Fat program, I opted for the simplest guideline for men, women, big, small, young, and old: *Drink 1 gallon of ice-cold water a day.*

Q: *Is it possible to drink too much cold water?*

A: Sure. Too much of almost any healthy practice can cause an eventual problem. In the medical literature, drinking too much water leads to a condition known as hyponatremia. Hyponatremia most often occurs in athletes involved in triathlons and ultramarathons. A few of these athletes consume many gallons of water during the course of these unusually long competitions, and because of the continuous activity they don't, or can't, stop to urinate. Thus, they impede their normal fluid-mineral balance and actually become intoxicated with too much water. Such a condition, however, is rare.

I've never observed anything close to intoxication happening with any of my Killing Fat participants, and some of them have consumed up to two gallons of water daily. Of course, they also have no trouble urinating frequently.

Note: Anyone with a kidney disorder, or taking diuretics, should consult a physician before trying superhydration.

Q: *I frequently read that slow fat loss, 1 to 2 pounds a week, is better for the body than fast fat loss, 4 to 5 pounds a week. What's the truth?*

A: I believe *fast* is best, given that what you lose is fat, not a lot of fluid. I like my aggressive six-week approach, as opposed to the long, slow, moderate styles. Why take six months to do something you can do in six weeks? Six weeks also keeps your momentum and enthusiasm at high levels.

The Killing Fat program is the fastest possible way to transfer fat out of your body. But please note, I did not say anything about fast fat loss being *easy*. It is not easy—it's very demanding.

Q: *You mentioned in part IV that keeping your body cool will help you burn more calories. Besides the cold plunge, do you have any additional tips for doing that?*

A: Yes, here are some practices that will assist you in losing more calories by staying cool.

- Dress cooler and lighter for work.
- Take off your coat sooner and keep it off longer.
- Select short sleeves more often.
- Don't wear a hat.
- Turn down the thermostat.
- Leave your socks at home, or go barefoot more often.
- Try to remain uncomfortably cool throughout the day and allow your skin's heating mechanism time to adjust.
- Negative-train in a cooler environment, if possible.
- Wear light, well-ventilated clothing when you exercise.

- Avoid sauna, steam, and whirlpool baths, as they cause excessive heat accumulation.
- Take cold showers after exercise.
- Place cold compresses on the back of your neck.
- Sleep cooler.
- Wean yourself from electric blankets and flannel sheets in the winter.

Q: *I'm into the cold plunge and your ideas on skin transfer of heat through conduction and radiation. What can I do to make my skin more efficient at getting rid of heat calories?*

A: Get leaner. Champion bodybuilders have known that for years. Your skin is very vascular. It is filled with arteries, capillaries, and veins. As you shrink your subcutaneous fat, the vessels in your skin will become more prevalent and more effective at eliminating heat. In short, you'll become more muscular and have more definition.

The cold plunge will help. Keep doing it at least three times a week. And so will negative strength training. There is no better way to condition your skin than working the underlying muscles. You can isolate almost any part of your body—from the little muscles of your feet and hands to the large muscles of your thighs and chest—that pumps blood to those specific areas. This surging blood brings nutrients and heat. The rising heat in the muscles must be released through the skin. And your skin learns to adapt better by becoming a more efficient heat regulator.

Q: *What about warming up before a negative-accentuated training session?*

A: There is some evidence to support the case for warming up as a safeguard against injury. Almost any sequence of light freehand movements can be used as a general warm-up to a vigorous strength-training routine. Suggested movements include head rotations, side bends, trunk twists, squats, and stationary cycling. A minute of each movement should be sufficient.

Q: *After a workout, should I cool down before taking a shower?*

A: Yes. After your last exercise is completed, you can cool down by walking around the training area, getting a drink of water, and moving your arms in slow circles. Continue these movements until your breathing has returned to normal and your heart rate has slowed. This usually takes 5 minutes.

Q: *When I do the sit-up on a declined bench or the abdominal crunch machine described in chapter 9, I feel it more in my upper abs. I need to work my lower abs. What exercise can I do for them?*

A: Both of those exercises work your lower abs, but you will never feel the effect in the lower area as much as you do in the upper region. Here are the reasons why.

First, the largest section of your abdominal muscles is high on your waist, under your rib cage—not low or beneath your navel. You almost always feel the abdominal exercises most in the mass of the muscles toward the origin.

Second, the long, paired rectus abdominis muscles originate under your rib cage and insert into your pelvis. But when these muscles get near the region of your navel, they actually plunge through an opening in the horizontally crossing transverse abdominis muscles. The transverse abdominis, which lies on top of the insertion point of the rectus abdominis, tends to reduce the sensitivity of the deeper rectus abdominis.

Third, sometimes bringing in the iliopsoas muscles—which connect to your spine and thigh bones and lie underneath the abdominal muscles—into action can synergize feeling in the region below your navel. If you are strong enough, you may want to try the hanging leg raise. The hanging leg raise involves hanging from an overhead bar and lifting your feet up smoothly and touching them to the bar and then lowering them slowly back to the bottom.

Fourth, many people confuse working their lower abs with the removal of fatty deposits below their navel. Remember, working the lower abs does not draw calories from fat that may lie near the involved muscles. Spot reduction of fat is a myth.

Q: *My body fat seems to be thickest over the sides of my waist. Can I ever get rid of these love handles?*

A: I understand what you are talking about. In chapter 15, Doug Spratt was correct when he noted that many men store fat first on the

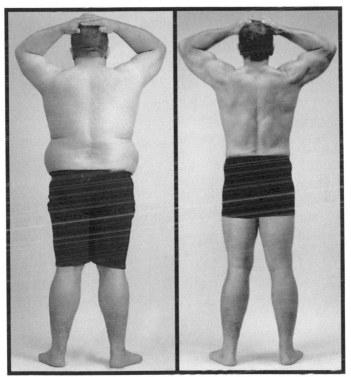

281.5 pounds   181 pounds

ANGEL RODRIGUEZ, age 48, height 5'8"
AFTER 30 WEEKS
121 pounds of fat loss
20.125 inches off waist
20.5 pounds of muscle gain

sides of their waist, which means it will be the last place the fat comes off. *First on, last off* is one of the basic principles of fat deposition and reduction.

I want you to look at the before-and-after photos of Angel Rodriguez on page 259. The time between the photos was thirty weeks. Rodriguez had some of the thickest love handles I've ever seen. And they did not start shrinking significantly until the fifteenth week. By the end of the thirtieth week—and after a reduction of 20 inches from his waist—his loves handles had absolutely disappeared.

Check out the muscularity of Rodriguez's back. He also added a bunch of solid muscle on his arms, shoulders, and upper and lower back. Building muscle at the same time as you are losing fat is a necessary part of the overall solution. (You'll also read more about Rodriguez's overall results in chapter 24.)

Yes, you can get rid of your love handles. Even if it takes you thirty weeks, you can do it.

Sure, you'll be challenged and tempted along the way. But you can combat each challenge and each temptation with discipline and patience.

You can conquer your love handles with Killing Fat.

Q: *My parents need less fat and more muscle. They are in their early eighties. Have you had any experience training people this age? Would you recommend that they try your program?*

A: Yes, I've trained a few women and men in this age group. A woman in her eighties who stands out in my mind is Nannette Carnes. In six weeks, she lost 12.5 pounds of fat and gained 1.5 pounds of muscle. Nannette, a former physical education teacher in Gainesville, was tall and poised. She never missed a workout, and she was a pleasure to train.

On the men's side, William R. "Bill" Kribs deserves more than a paragraph. Bill owns the gated community in Orlando where my family and I lived for fifteen years. In 2013, he joined my Intensive Coaching course, which I direct out of my home gym. Bill lived 300 yards

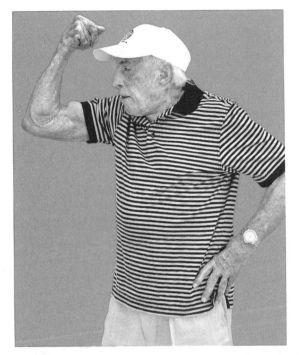

Bill Kribs, at 5'9" tall and a weight of 158 pounds, has a body-fat level of 14.5 percent, which is incredible for his age. And how about that peak on his right biceps?

from me and he bicycled down to train two mornings a week. Gradually, he chipped away at his fat and muscle.

In nine months, he lost 10.8 pounds of fat and also built 12.35 pounds of muscle. His favorite exercises were the leg press and the dumbbell curl. For six years and counting, Bill has locked in and maintained his 158-pound condition.

One highlight of his transformation: In 2016, his daughter, Karen, became concerned about her dad's forgetfulness. She made an appointment for him to undergo a complete physical and mental evaluation by Orlando Health's Center for Aging. After three days of very thorough testing, the doctors concluded that William R. Kribs was perfectly healthy . . . for a seventy-year-old man.

"That's great"—Bill smiled—"but you know what? I just celebrated my birthday: number ninety-six."

Bill has now reduced his workouts from twice a week to once a week . . . and he's always at my home gym on Tuesday mornings at ten a.m. Muscular strength is extremely important to Bill, who will turn one hundred years old in 2020. Bill is determined to live longer stronger. He's my kind of guy, and he remains one of my best friends.

I'm twenty-four years younger than Bill . . . and this man *inspires me to train harder.*

Back to the question: Yes, your parents can progress through my Killing Fat program. But it's essential that they obtain their physician's okay before they get started. Get a copy of this book for your parents to take on their consult so the doctor can understand what's in store for them.

Q: *I'm not into exercising. Is it okay to use the recommended Killing Fat diet without the 30–10–30 training?*

A: The Killing Fat eating plan without negative-accentuated exercise does result in weight loss. But at least 25 percent and as much as 40 percent of the weight loss comes not from body fat, but from the muscles, vital organs, and fluid.

Loss of proteins and fluids from these vital cells is difficult to avoid with even a small reduction in the calorie intake of an inactive person. The problem is readily overcome if a descending-calorie diet is combined with negative-accentuated strength training.

I would not recommend that you try the diet without the strength training. Once you lost your desired amount of weight, you would surely gain it back and then some. The goal of Killing Fat is not only to lose weight, but also to make sure that the weight you lose is fat.

Adding muscular pounds to your body efficiently with 30–10–30 is the best way to be certain that the weight you lose is from your body's fat stores. And increasing your muscle mass is one of the best ways to keep the fat off permanently.

Proper strength training and 30–10–30 have a lot to offer your body.

Q: *In chapter 2, you stated that only 17 percent of your test panelists from Gainesville Health & Fitness had kept their lost fat off after three years. Aren't you discouraged by that low number?*

A: I'm not discouraged, but I am certainly concerned. I do think the number is actually higher than that because the population in Gainesville is so mobile. Approximately 125,000 people live in Gainesville. Some 55,000 are students who go to the University of Florida and another 16,000 are enrolled at nearby Santa Fe Community College. Plus, there are 30,000 older professionals in Gainesville who work for or with one or the other of these institutions. Thus, many of these people move out of the area and change addresses, get married or divorced, discontinue their fitness memberships, or simply don't answer emails and questionnaires.

Even if my success rate were three times 17 percent, or 51 percent, I'd still be frustrated. I want every man and woman who progresses through my programs to *master* how to keep their lost fat off permanently. That is my ongoing goal.

But if you think 17 percent is a discouraging success rate, how about the more typical 1 percent success rate? That includes Jenny Craig, Weight Watchers, Nutrisystem, Volumetrics Diet, *Biggest Loser Diet*, SlimFast diet, Atkins, South Beach, and the diets recommended in popular weight loss books such as *Wheat Belly*, *Grain Brain*, and *The Bulletproof Diet*. And then there's all kinds of related materials on ketogenic, or "keto," dieting. You don't have much of a chance at long-term success on any of them.

If you need to get rid of excessive fat, I invite and challenge you to get started on Killing Fat today.

PATIENCE AND OVERLEARNING

KEY PRACTICES FOR MAINTENANCE

PATIENCE IS THE ability to endure without complaint. It allows you to stick to a task until completion.

It takes patience to transform your body: to kill the fat, destroy the flab, shrink the stomach, build the muscles—and most important—maintain those results permanently.

Patience, like any other quality, must be learned. But how long does it take to become patient?

To help answer this question, I've gathered some related facts while working with thousands of overfat people, especially from observing the successful compared to the unsuccessful. From fifty years of study, the single most relevant fact I've observed that helps people maintain results is *overlearning*.

Overlearning and Winning

Overlearning means practice beyond goal achievement. Seldom does a serious-minded athlete ever practice enough. Steph Curry, the All-

Pro scoring champion for the NBA's Golden State Warriors, is sure that he has shot the ball at the basket—not thousands of times—millions of times! Overlearning is one reason Curry is such a superior shooter.

Overlearning as it relates to the Killing Fat program means the practicing of certain behaviors again and again until they are so ingrained that almost nothing can disturb them. Overlearning produces automatic actions. Without thinking, you respond with the correct behavior. The more times you experience the desired response, the better you get and the more lasting the pattern becomes.

Of the thousands of people who have successfully finished my fat-loss programs, the ones who have kept the fat off have done so because of overlearning. The salient rules—such as eat smaller meals, superhydrate your system, and keep your muscles strong—have been internalized.

How long does it take to overlearn and internalize?

21 Days and 100 Days

I've observed with my test panelists that it takes approximately twenty-one days to establish a pattern and one hundred days to make that pattern automatic. In other words, the Killing Fat program gets easier for most people after three weeks. If they continue the plan for three months, their daily actions become almost automatic.

Be aware, too, that many psychologists believe that hundred-day time frame means one hundred *consecutive* days. If you practice the discipline for sixty-two days and break the pattern on day 63, you must start over. Maybe that's why it's so hard for many people to keep the fat off permanently.

Yet I've seen many people succeed. One person who stands out in my mind is Storm Roberts.

Storm Roberts: A Big-Time Loser

Storm Roberts was in one of the test groups that went through the program at Gainesville Health & Fitness in the spring of 2013. Roberts is a well-known morning-show host on 98.5 KTK in the Gainesville area. After he went through his first strength-training routine, two things were obvious to me. One, Roberts had the biggest belly in the entire group. At a body weight of 256.86 pounds, his waist measured 46.375 inches at the navel. Two, Roberts quickly mastered the negative-accentuated training style in his very first workout.

At the end of three weeks, it was evident that Roberts was really into the program. He'd lost at least a pound each day. During the initial six weeks, he dropped 38.2 pounds of fat. Then he shed 19 pounds over a second six weeks, and a final 8.47 pounds during a third six-week phase. Over fifteen weeks, Roberts lost 65.67 pounds of fat and 9.5 inches off his waist. Plus, he built 11.81 pounds of solid muscle.

From 2014 through 2017, on my numerous visits to Gainesville Health & Fitness, I would often see Roberts. He was usually answering the questions of folks who were going through the Killing Fat program for their first six weeks. Storm was well liked at the fitness center and generally all over Gainesville. Plus, I kept noticing that he was always in tip-top shape—*always*.

It's been almost five years since Roberts dropped 65 pounds of fat. How was he able to keep his physique in such lean condition? That's how I started my conversation with him on February 20, 2018.

Getting Control

"Getting control of my diet was the biggest breakthrough for me," Roberts said to me as we settled in for a conversation near the smoothie bar at Gainesville Health & Fitness. Roberts is on early-morning radio

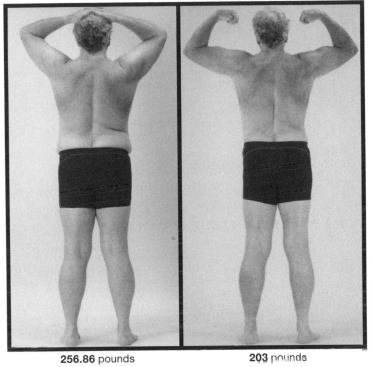

256.86 pounds   203 pounds

STORM ROBERTS, age 61, height 6'0"
AFTER 15 WEEKS
65.67 pounds of fat loss
9.5 inches off waist
11.81 pounds of muscle gain

five days a week and he's off the air at ten a.m. Later, on Mondays, Wednesdays, and Fridays, he usually goes to the fitness center.

"I love to cook," Roberts continued, "and I have the luxury of planning and shopping for meals. Over the last four years, I've become a food snob. For my continued leanness, there are certain foods I will not allow into my body."

"Okay, Storm, I hear what you're saying," I replied, "but give me a few examples."

"Fast foods—like you see in McDonald's, Burger King, and Wendy's," Roberts said. "Any food fried—no, no, no. I've lost my taste for them and don't even like hamburgers anymore. I find myself migrating to a more plant-based diet, and I have come up with some delicious recipes."

"Yes, I like the plant-based foods, too," I noted. "But I also must admit that I like an occasional Burger King Whopper Jr. or a Subway Cold Cut Combo with plenty of fresh veggies. Storm, besides avoiding fast foods, do you have a maintenance formula that you could share with my *Killing Fat* readers?"

"Sure, here's what I do each day . . ."

Storm's Maintenance Formula

- Eat approximately the same breakfast and lunch. Each small meal is 400 calories.
- Select and bag my snacks for the day, which are usually apples and nuts.
- Review my carb-to-fat-to-protein ratios on my iPad with the MyPlate tracker from LIVESTRONG.
- Make a preliminary list of what I am going to eat for the rest of the day.
- Maintain my 50–25–25 ratio of carbs to fat to protein by looking ahead and making various additions and subtractions.
- Prepare my evening meal, with any adjustments.

"The LiveStrong.com website shows a pie chart with the carb/fat/protein breakdown so I can nail the numbers within a few percentage points every day. It's sort of like a video game that I win every time I play.

"Sipping ice water throughout the day, the negative resistance training twice a week, and my nightly walking have also been important factors. Not only have I maintained my excessive fat loss, I've halved my blood pressure medicine. Overall, my life has taken on new meaning."

"Storm," I asked, "what about the hundred-day continuation and warning that I stressed to your initial group of test panelists? Did that ring a bell with you?"

After 100 Days: Taking Charge

"Yes, it did," Roberts replied. "Going back to 2013, after one hundred consecutive days of being strict, my body automated to the new routine and I didn't have to write things down as often. Now I have my way of eating and cooking that are a huge lifestyle change, and I'm more comfortable with this Storm Roberts.

"Five years ago, I weighed more than 250 pounds. The best thing is that I'm 56 pounds lighter . . . and the new Storm Roberts has taken charge. It used to be the other way around. The food and the social environment dominated me. Not anymore.

"It feels great to take charge and be in control."

Just Say NO!

"That's terrific, Storm," I said "You are certainly an inspiration to many members of Gainesville Health & Fitness and to your radio audience. How about a final thought for my *Killing Fat* readers?"

Storm settled into a quiet mood for several moments, then said:

"I still have to fight the little man who lives in my head. He thinks I need more food than I really do. He begs me to stop and have a doughnut. He provokes my memory of prime rib and horseradish cream sauce. I fight him every day.

"But I end up winning . . . and then . . . smirking. Why? Because I hit that little man repeatedly with the strongest word in the language. That word is *NO*."

"I like that lesson." I smiled. "After four years of dealing with that little man in your head, does it get easier and easier to tell him *no*?"

"Yes, it does," Storm noted. "The whiff of hot doughnuts, or the aroma of prime rib on the grill, is much less now than it was several years ago. I think he will become less and less and finally disappear as I get even more control."

"In other words," I chimed in, "eventually you'll kill and bury that little man."

We both did a fast fist bump, laughed, and repeated in unison: *"KILLING FAT."*

"Thank you, Storm," I said. "I appreciate what you've achieved and your generosity in sharing your experiences."

Practice and More Practice

Important: Before Storm Roberts could say he was in control, he had to overlearn his daily rituals. In Roberts's case, it took him fifteen weeks, or 105 days—which is slightly longer than the hundred days I mentioned earlier. But remember also that Roberts had to lose 65 pounds of fat to reach his goal, which is double what most guys have as an initial objective.

With people who need to lose 25 to 30 pounds, one hundred days becomes an overlearning target. But my experience in dealing with thousands of people reveals that two hundred days is better than one hundred. Within reason, more is better.

Specific Maintenance Guidelines for Killing Fat

Successful maintenance, like successful overlearning, requires a continuation of the practices that you've been adhering to for the last several months. There are, however, a few minor adjustments that you must understand and apply.

Follow a carbohydrate-rich moderate-calorie eating plan: Carbohydrate-rich meals are still what you should be consuming, but your total calories per day can be increased. Generally, a young man of average height and weight should be able to maintain his body weight on 2,000 to 2,600 calories a day. An average young woman would require from 1,500 to 2,200 calories per day.

You can figure out your maintenance level by gradually adding calories back into your eating plan. A man should start with 2,000 calories a day. A woman should try 1,500 a day. Stay at that level for a week. If you are still losing weight, raise the level by 100 calories a day for the next week. In another week or two, your body weight will stabilize. You'll then know that you've reached the upper limit to your maintenance calorie level.

Eat smaller meals more frequently: You've been limiting your six small meals per day to 300 to 400 calories or fewer. To maintain your body weight, set the limit to 500 calories for a man and 400 calories for a woman. Sometimes a few extra calories is acceptable. But anything more than 600 calories in a meal means your body will store the excess in your fat cells. Be careful.

Superhydrate with 1 gallon of cold water each day: You've experienced the positive effects of sipping plenty of ice-cold water. You should now understand the importance of superhydration in fat loss, muscle building, skin health, and internal and external cooling. Water supports almost all your functions. Make superhydration a permanent part of your new lifestyle.

Strength train once a week: If you've mastered the 30–10–30 style of strength training, then once a week is going to work fine for you. Some of my best trainees, however, still like to strength train with 8 to 12 reps performed in a normal manner. If that's your mind-set, then twice a week is probably better than once a week. Or you might explore going three times in two weeks and doing two normal routines and one 30–10–30.

Keep in mind that more strength training is not better. Better strength training is harder. Apply this concept consistently, and your muscularity and overall leanness may well exceed your goals.

Practice a few other actions, as needed: Any of the other guidelines—such as extra sleep, the cold plunge, and staying cool—can be reinstated into your maintenance schedule anytime you need a synergistic boost.

Back to Patience

The title *Killing Fat* does not exactly stress the value of patience. As you may realize by now, however, patience is an important aspect of the entire system.

Storm Roberts and the others whose success stories you've read about in this book have all learned plenty about patience in their personal journeys to rid their bodies of excess fat.

As I said in the introduction, losing pounds and inches of fat from your body requires discipline. The entire process demands hard work.

But because of the repeated hard work, it does, in a sense, get less complicated. It gets less complicated because the course teaches you to endure without complaint. And in the process, you perfect your patience.

Yes, patience is truly a virtue. And you've got it!

CONSIDERATIONS FOR A BETTER LIFE

Here are nine actions, which have not been covered in this book, that will help you better your life.

ADD A TWIST TO YOUR NEXT PB&J

The twist comes by way of Buffalo Bills strength-training coach Will Greenberg. During preseason practices, the Bills' cafeteria prepares meals and snacks for a hundred professional football players, some of whom weigh more than 300 pounds. Greenberg works with a nutritionist to set the cafeteria menus.

By far the most popular snack is a peanut butter and jelly

sandwich, and the twist comes from using Ezekiel bread. Two slices of Ezekiel bread contain 160 calories, and the bread is loaded with healthy seeds, grains, and sprouts. The Bills like jam instead of jelly, because jam is made from whole fruit, while jelly is made from only the juice of the fruit. A lot of the guys also prefer Smucker's Organic Peanut Butter.

One PB&J prepared with the above ingredients contains approximately 400 calories—and some of the guys consume three or four a day between their normal meals. Cut the sandwich in half, and you have two Killing Fat snacks. Enjoy.

SURROUND YOURSELF WITH LIKE-MINDED PEOPLE

To maintain your fat loss, studies show that if one spouse became obese, the likelihood that the other spouse would also become obese increased by 37 percent. Another study found that participants with at least one successful weight loss partner dropped significantly more weight than those with no successful partners.

KEEP YOUR KITCHEN CLEAN

Some three thousand people die from food poisoning each year in the United States. Even common foods like berries, cantaloupe, sprouts, and chicken can make you sick or even kill you. Your action plan: Keep your kitchen pristine, wash your hands and utensils before and after handling food, separate raw and cooked foods, and refrigerate perishable food promptly.

SAVE YOUR DOLLARS

Money might not make you happier, but it will help you live longer. Stanford researchers found in 2016 that people whose income was in the top 1 percent lived nearly fifteen years longer than those in the bottom 1 percent. The disparity was attributed to heathier behaviors in high-income groups, including less smoking and lower obesity levels.

GET A DOG

Studies have found that owning a pet can reduce anxiety, lower blood pressure, and even improve the odds of surviving a heart attack. A recent study in Sweden recommends owning a dog. Dog owners are more likely to be physically active and are less vulnerable to the effects of hormones related to stress.

LAUGH, A LOT

Laughter really is positive medicine. Studies show that laughter reduces stress, boosts the immune system, reduces pain, and improves blood flow to the brain.

TRY TO STAY OUT OF THE HOSPITAL

Here's something to consider: A 2016 study at Johns Hopkins University found that 250,000 patients die each year in hospitals from misdiagnoses, poor conditions, incorrect practices, and drug errors. Perhaps the best way to avoid a grave condition is not to enter the system at all.

GET MARRIED

The Framingham Offspring Study found that married men had a 46 percent lower risk of death than never-married men. A 2014 study by New York University's Langone Medical Center revealed that married men and women had a 5 percent lower risk of cardiovascular disease.

READ MORE BOOKS

Research at Yale University supports the longevity benefits of reading. Newspapers and magazines, as well as material on the internet, will work—but books proved best. People who read books for as little as 30 minutes a day had a significant survival advantage over those who were not page turners.

23

JEFF SHAW'S REPORT

HIS KILLING FAT JOURNEY

ONCE IN EACH decade of adulthood, if you are lucky, you work with a person who not only grasps what you are trying to teach, but who takes the concept several steps farther than you antici pated. That's exactly what Jeff Shaw of Leicester, England, did with me in 2016 and 2017.

Since Shaw is a precise record-keeper, I asked him to look back and assemble a report of his body's transformation from fatness to leanness.

Meeting Ellington

It's mid-February and inevitably it's cold and it's raining. I'm hoping it doesn't snow, because today I'm flying from London, England, to Orlando, Florida, to spend a whole day with Ellington Darden—a man I've spoken to for less than 15 minutes on the phone but whose books on bodybuilding and nutrition I've been reading for thirty years.

I've been strength training since I was eleven years old. I used to compete in bodybuilding contests. Now I'm fifty-five, but, sadly,

I don't display the physique of someone who has put well over forty years in at the gym. I first read one of Ellington's books when I was in my late twenties. It set me on a successful path, and I've used many of the training methods he has outlined to add muscle. I know that because I'm big, at around 224 pounds at a height of 5 feet 10 inches.

My problem is that I'm also overfat and have become increasingly unhappy with my shape and my apparent lack of ability to rid myself of that flab as I grow older. I'm no stranger to diets and have followed several to the letter. Yet I'm still out of shape and I can't figure out why. Meeting Dr. Darden face-to-face and discussing where I'm going wrong has become close to an obsession. There must be something complex I'm not doing or am missing. My frustration with my condition is at a peak.

I arrive safely in Orlando and visit Ellington's home gym the next day.

The Weigh-In, Photos, and Workout

"You have this really funny accent." I smile. Ellington glances up. "I've got a funny accent? I'm thinking *you've* got a weird one," he says with a grin. We're getting to know each other and swapping bodybuilding anecdotes. Slowly we move on to the more serious stuff of why I'm here.

I strip to my gray training shorts and we do circumference and body-fat measurements. I'm a few pounds down from what I normally weigh. Ellington tells me I've got some good thighs and calves and some muscular triceps as well. Secretly, I'm pleased, but use the opportunity to bemoan my lack of bodybuilding success—I've never won a contest—blaming my genetics. Without saying it, I'm trying to blame being fat on my genetics as well, rather than anything I've done or any mistakes I've made.

Then we prepare for photos. I take off my glasses and shuffle barefoot out in front of his garage. I can't see without them, but I'm conscious of how far out my tummy is sticking. I concentrate on playing hide and seek with his dog. I don't like dogs, but he seems to like licking my bare legs. I wonder if he's trying to eat me. The game continues as Ellington snaps the photos. It removes my mind from how fat I really am.

Time to really begin now. I shuffle back to his private gym and re-dress into my bright yellow top. I'm determined to show him I might be fat but I know what I'm doing in the gym.

I'm pushed through eight upper-body exercises. We use a 15-second negative, 15-second positive, 15-second negative, followed by 8 to 10 normal reps, for most of the workout. I am used to exercising hard and to the style of training we use. I have, after all, read the books. About three-quarters of the way through, Ellington admonishes me as I fail on a shoulder press. "C'mon, Jeff, you're stronger than this. Let's go!"

I'm not. This really is it. I'm not holding back. I'm puffing and blowing. Again—this is something I'm entirely used to. Ellington asks me if I'm okay to train my legs. "Oh yeah," I respond as enthusiastically as I can. I am determined not to show any signs of weakness.

30–10–30, the Knock-Out, Carbohydrates, and *Killing Fat*

"Jeff, I want you to try 30–10–30 on the legs," Ellington says. "It's my latest method of negative-accentuated training." He explains what I need to do, and after one set of the calf raise and one set of the leg press, I'm thinking that this new negative style is the absolute best for growth stimulation that I've ever felt.

I finish the workout and we sit down to chat. I'm breathless and my fingers are tingling a bit. The feeling gets worse. My whole body is now tingling. I go as green as Ellington's top. "You're getting too much oxygen," he drawls. I end up lying facedown on the cool floor and breathing in and out of a paper bag. Getting my own carbon dioxide into my system tells my body that having too much oxygen is not going to damage me. Ten minutes later I start to feel more normal.

"You have to tell me," says Ellington when I'm finally able to sit upright again, "what do you want most from me?"

"I'm definitely going to take 30–10–30 back to England and apply it," I reply. "But it's my diet that I can't seem to get right."

Ellington asks me for a list of what I'm eating. I'm less than half-way through reciting my typical high-protein bodybuilding regime when he stops me. "Where are your carbohydrates?" he challenges, his face a bit flushed. "Jeff, you're not serious about this!"

My heart flutters and a lot of unsavory words form in the back of my head. I keep quiet, but I know I'm looking glum.

The interrogation continues: "Have you read *The Body Fat Break-through*? Why aren't you following the diet in that book?"

Good question. It's about time I did. After all, that's what I'm here for. All other diets have failed me.

Ellington goes over some helpful dietary guidelines with me and tells me about his new book project, which he wants to call *Killing Fat*. The book will unveil his 30–10–30 knock-out punch. Seems I've already been down, almost cold, for that count.

Killing Fat. That's exactly what I want to do, and I say that to Ellington. He cracks a slight smile, sort of the way Clint Eastwood used to do in those spaghetti westerns.

My Progress After 2 Weeks: Minus 8.5 Pounds

The first day I arrive back home, I locate my copy of *The Body Fat Breakthrough* and pore over the diet plans. They are so simple. Why didn't I just follow them? I write down everything I need to make this plan a success, drive to the supermarket, and fill my shopping cart.

I am less concerned about the workout plans in the book, as I know I am quite capable of writing and undertaking my own routines that are completely aligned to the principles laid out by Dr. Darden, including a few performed 30–10–30. I even send him a copy of all my future workouts for some sort of verification and am pleased when I get the virtual thumbs-up. The plan is that I train only once per week on around eight exercises. That's about 20 minutes a week.

I start on the diet that same day. I'm used to sticking to a diet. Planning, preparing, having everything at hand is not new. But Ellington has told me in no uncertain terms that I've been following the wrong one.

"Once a week? For twenty minutes?" Andy at work laughs when I tell him the exercise plan. "You need a lot more exercise to get rid of that," he says with scorn as he points at my bulging tummy.

Two weeks of diet and exercise later, I'm sitting at home and writing down what I weigh. I've weighed myself three times. I can't quite believe it. I have lost an amazing 8.5 pounds. From two weeks and only two workouts in the gym, I've lost more than I have ever lost on any other plan. I'm stunned with my level of success. Andy isn't going to like this.

After 4 Weeks: Minus 14.25 Pounds

No one at work has really noticed any changes in me. Andy is being really quiet. I'm an engineer for a large automotive company. My work is stressful and demanding at times. I'm also the caretaker for my elderly mum, which is equally stressful and demanding. I've decreased my calories and I'm on the edge of hunger all the time, feeling cold, spending time in the bathroom, and am disappointed that no one at work has said anything positive because I have now lost an additional 5.75 pounds.

I need a bit of that positive reinforcement. Despite my melancholy, the actual food plan, the gym, and the workouts are really no problem at all. I may be hungry, but the diet is easy to follow and I'm doing it. I really enjoy working out as well—who would stick to a pastime for over forty years if they didn't enjoy it? You have to be resilient to train the way Dr. Darden asks you to. I'm sure younger men would relish the challenge. I do, too. No exercise, routine, or amount of effort fazes me, but I really don't know why I can't bring myself to walk as much as I'm supposed to. It's a real challenge for me. I write an email.

> Hi Ellington,
> Well, after 4 weeks I'm pleased to say I'm down to 207 pounds. Still sticking 100 percent with everything diet and water wise. Sleep is around 9½ hours a night as a minimum.
> My waist is now: 40¾ inches above navel, 40¾ inches at navel and 38½ inches below navel. Currently on 1400 calories per day.

A reply comes straight back.

> Way to go Jeff,
> Sounds like everything is going great. How's your level of hunger each day? If there are no significant problems, I'd say go ahead and lower your daily calories to 1,300 per day for the following two weeks. That's probably as low as you need to go. The inches you are losing around your waist are adding up nicely. Again, stay strict.

I am rejuvenated by this. We all need positive reinforcement at times. I make up my mind to seek out people who are going to give me that on a regular basis. I also get serious about this walking once and for all. I can hear Ellington's Texan drawl telling me over and over, *You're not serious about this*. I use it to put fire in my belly. I'm not giving in.

After 6 Weeks: Minus 19.25 Pounds

I have now lost 19.25 pounds since I began, and I look like a different man. People at work are now looking at me strangely, like they know something has changed but they don't quite know what. There's a few polite "have you lost weight queries" going on. I am over the moon, and my excitement is showing. I sit next to 260-pound Tony at work. He tells me he's inspired to start dieting. I tell him to buy Darden's books.

After 8 Weeks: Minus 23 Pounds

Another two weeks, and I'm down to just under 198 pounds. Everything is now going exceptionally well. I am so delighted by my progress that absolutely nothing and nobody is going to stop me now. I even have to lead the delivery of a two-day technical engineering seminar. I'm on my feet for nine hours both days. I'm tired, but I stick to it.

I knew well in advance that I have the seminar approaching. It's a careful balancing act, but I am able to prepare all my food in advance. With some careful planning and thought, I even manage to tailor the breaks in the seminar so I can eat at the right times. I sip my water all day long, although finding time to run to the toilet does prove to be a bit of a challenge. I sleep extraordinarily well both nights.

I have also been working hard in the gym. In total I'm dieting, eating, sleeping, walking, and drinking water to the letter. I'm even putting a cold compress on the back of my neck three times a week. It's pretty uncomfortable and I dread it a little bit, but this isn't about a nice, easy process. This is about hard work. This is about driving for success. My discipline from all those years of bodybuilding is proving useful.

I'm finding that alternating workout cadences in the gym is giving me additional little challenges that I am relishing, and I have been alternating workout styles mostly between using an exercise cadence of 30–10–30 one week and one of 15–15–15, plus 8 to 12 repetitions, with a couple of exercises done 30–30–30 thrown in. From time to time I pick a weight that is too heavy for 30–30–30 (for some reason, I never seem to pick a weight that's too light).

After 10 Weeks: Minus 28 Pounds

I am down another 5 pounds. My total weight loss is a tad over 28 pounds in ten weeks. I write to Dr. Darden again: Could I lose weight even more quickly? "Don't do anything foolish," he warns. "You've got a lot of determination. You've disciplined yourself to stick to a program exactly as specified for ten weeks." And I have. The results show. Just stick to the plan. That's all I need to do.

My trousers are far too big in the waist. Martin, at work, looks at me with bug eyes. "You have got to stop losing weight," he chides. Tony keeps looking at Dr. Darden's books on Amazon.com. Others are finally noticing. Even Andy is being a bit more cautious in his criticism. It's not surprising. I look very different now.

A few others are being just as negative as Andy was, but most are asking what I've done, and how easy is it. One person is going around telling everyone that Jeff is on the "high-carb diet." No. I'm not. I'm on a sensible, balanced diet. Probably for the first time in my life.

Caroline is asking me why I don't eat more protein. She's a long-distance runner. I tell her our bodies don't need it and we use carbohydrates as our primary source of fuel for exercise and recovery. She shakes her head warily. We agree to disagree. There's not a chance I'm going back to that. No more high-protein bodybuilding-magazine stuff for me. What's more, I know I'm not finished yet.

After 12 Weeks: Minus 33.5 Pounds

I'm there. As a result of eleven workouts, totaling 195 minutes, and twelve weeks of dieting, I'm now at 187.75 pounds, for a total loss of 33.5 pounds. Originally, Ellington challenged me to lose 25 pounds, so I've exceeded that by 8.5 pounds.

I roughly calculate that I am now at 9.3 percent body fat. Bearing in mind that I knew how to train and had already used the workout

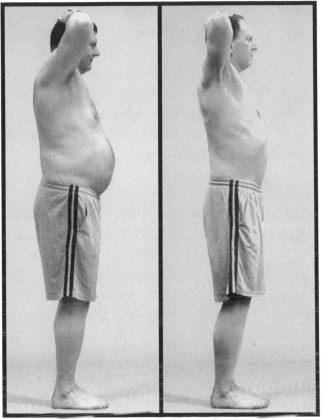

221.5 pounds   1/7.75 pounds

JEFF SHAW, age 55, height 5'9.75"
AFTER 18 WEEKS
53.75 pounds of fat loss
8 inches off waist
10 pounds of muscle gain

principles devised by Dr. Darden, nothing has really changed in that department. The only differences for me are how I eat and the deliberate steps I now take, to use Ellington's words, to "lose body heat to the environment." I seriously can't believe the difference between getting the diet wrong, i.e., getting fat and staying fat, and getting the diet right. Andy offers me a bit of cake to celebrate.

The first two weeks I lost the most rapidly, and the losses have been steady at about 2 to 2.25 pounds a week since then. Surprisingly, after an initial quick drop, my waist measurements have not changed much for quite a while and are now at 37.5 inches above the navel, 37.5 inches at the navel, and 37.5 inches below the navel. That's a drop of 7.625 inches from my waist. I'd like a smaller waist, but I have to accept that belly fat will always be with me to a certain extent. I wish I was younger. I'm sure my waist would be tighter. I can honestly blame genetics now. I can live with that—just!

After 18 Weeks: Minus 43 Pounds of Weight and *53 Pounds of Fat*

I'm not finished yet. Ellington has given me another target. He wants me to go for six more weeks and lose another 7 pounds. I respond to this immediately: I'm completely committed. I know exactly what to do. It's another calorie descent. By the time I've finished in late June, I weigh 177.75 pounds. I've beaten his target by almost 3 pounds.

In a recent email, Ellington reminded me that I had been talking about weight loss and not fat loss. I had reduced my body weight by 43 pounds, but I needed to add my muscle gain, which was a solid 10 pounds, to the weight loss to determine my total fat loss.

In total, I've disposed of 53 pounds of fat. That's right: *53 pounds*. I'm elated.

The Long Haul

Twenty months have passed since that first meeting with Ellington. I've had to buy all new clothes, and I'm "styling" and looking younger than normal at my fifty-seven years. Andy retired and has moved on, Tony has read several of Ellington's books and is now cutting calories and drinking ice water, and even Caroline is eating more carbohydrates.

The lean, strong Jeff Shaw is front and center. And I'm spreading the word about *Killing Fat*.

Most of all, I'm living it: Now, and for the long haul.

P.S.: Basic Principles

Six weeks have slipped by since I finished writing my journal. I was determined to carry on. Progress has been so good over the last two years, and I am so happy with what I've achieved that I didn't want any breaks or disruptions. Ellington has reinforced to me several times that it's not just a short-term plan that I've followed. It's a plan for the future as well.

If only life were like that.

My new challenge has been an overnight and quite severe deterioration of my mum's health. She's been hospitalized, and as her caretaker, this has derailed any thoughts of my continuing to train or stick to a structured diet plan . . . until the future is a bit clearer.

To take my mind off my troubles, I've been reflecting on the basic principles behind my muscular results. I decided to visualize them in a triangle, as shown below.

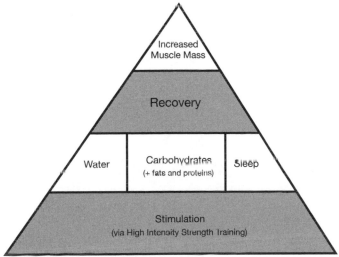

©Jeffrey E Shaw December 2017

The principles are based on the primary aim of increasing muscle, or, as Ellington has noted repeatedly, "building muscle for losing fat." More muscle is better for overall health and plays a significant role in maintenance due to its high metabolic demand.

The basic principles in the triangle, starting at the bottom, are as follows:

1. Brief stimulation through negative-accentuated strength training
2. Correct nutrition—primarily water, carbohydrates, fats, and proteins—plus extra sleep
3. Adequate recovery, measured in days, to allow the stimulus and nutrition to be effective

Combined together, the result was that I increased my muscle mass by 10 pounds.

Yes, putting on 10 pounds of muscle was a goal I was pleased to achieve. But I'm equally pleased to understand that the entire process begins at the bottom-floor level of *stimulation*—stimulation from hard, progressive, negative-accentuated training.

Without such stimulation, my fat loss would have probably been significantly reduced by at least 50 percent—from 53 pounds to 26.5 pounds.

After forty years of lifting weights, it's about time I learned how to achieve efficient results. I hope my triangle graphic can help you kill your fat, too.

24

MY CHAMPIONS

THE BEST OF THE BEST

THIS CHAPTER SHOWCASES my male trainees who have achieved what I judge to be the best overall results in two categories: 6 weeks and longer than 6 weeks. More than 700 men were considered. I also have a category for those men interested only in developing muscular size quickly.

In my selection of a champion, I do not use total fat loss as the single indicator of the winner. I take into account age, height, weight, fat loss, inches lost, muscle gain, and improvement from before to after photos. Fat loss to height is also considered, because taller individuals have an advantage, as their height is more effective at transferring heat as compared to shorter people.

Here are my champions.

Drumroll please . . .

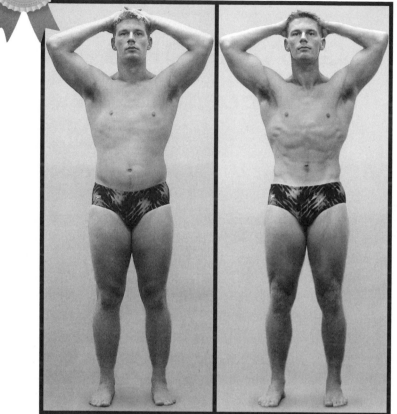

223.75 pounds   192 pounds

TOM WYKLE, age 28, height 6'1"
AFTER 6 WEEKS
fat loss **35.5** pounds
muscle gain **3.75** pounds

Tom Wykle: In 1998, when I met Tom Wykle, he was a professional water skier at SeaWorld Orlando. I thought he would perform much better if he lost 20 pounds of fat, so I challenged him to do that. He not only did that, but more, in six weeks. In his "after" photo, Tom shows a 32-inch waist and an etched six-pack. Today, he's a firefighter and EMT in Orlando, where he has been employed for fourteen years.

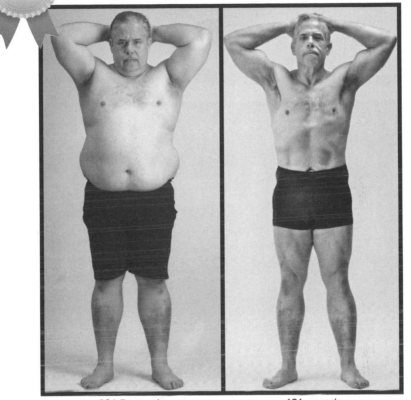

281.5 pounds   **181** pounds

ANGEL RODRIGUEZ, age 48, height 5'8"
AFTER 30 WEEKS
fat loss **121** pounds
muscle gain **20.5** pounds

Angel Rodriguez: Of the 1,209 individuals I've trained at Gainesville Health & Fitness, eleven weighed more than 300 pounds. But none of those 300-pounders ever lost more fat than Angel Rodriguez. Angel, at a starting body weight of 281.5 pounds, lost 121 pounds of fat. Can you imagine dropping 20 inches off your waist? That's exactly what Angel did. His workouts were amazing, as he is extremely strong and it shows throughout his body. He built 20.5 pounds of solid muscle.

Angel is a friend to all, including those with four legs, as he is the most recognized and popular animal-control officer in Gainesville and Alachua County.

Muscle Building in 2 Weeks

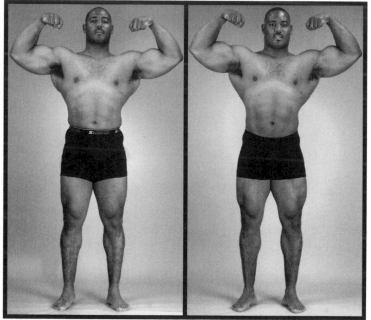

234.75 pounds   238 pounds

EDWIN "TRUCK" BROWN, age 43, height 5'10"
AFTER 2 WEEKS
fat loss **9.46** pounds
muscle gain **12.71** pounds

Edwin "Truck" Brown: There are several hundred bodybuilders at Gainesville Health & Fitness. By far the most popular one is a man known affectionately as "Truck." In the summer of 2012, I selected five bodybuilders to go through a special two-week big-arm program. These guys were trained twice a week on one set of eight negative-accentuated exercises. Brown performed the best, adding

12.71 pounds of muscle. His already massive arms grew by more than an inch. His contracted left upper arm, in an unpumped cold condition, measured 20.125 inches. "I started training in high school," Brown said, "but my arms have never been so big." *Important:* Brown was not on growth drugs. And he has not entered a physique contest in fifteen years. During the hours the sun is shining, Brown is in the landscape and pest-control businesses in Gainesville. But at night, you can usually find him training at the fitness center, where his persona is the size of a truck . . . a big truck.

A Future Fat-Fighting Team

A wise colleague once told me, "It's not whether you *win* or *lose* that counts, it's how you *LOOK* when you cross the finish line." Of course, your health is also important. But never underestimate the power of your physical appearance.

You can help. Get your body lean, strong, and good-looking with *Killing Fat*. Gladly share your success and how-to with your friends, and especially those you love. Together, we can blast belly bloat, build muscle, and kill fat.

KILLING FAT AND THE MIX

THE QUEST FOR THERMODYNAMIC SYNERGY

AS I LOOK back over my half century of working with overfat and out-of-shape people, I can remember often being asked:

What's the single most important factor in getting a lean, strong body for life?

Over five decades, my answers have broadened. Initially, I would have said a reduced-calorie diet. Later, a reduced-calorie, carbohydrate-rich diet. Later still, I would have brought in the importance of strength training. After that, I would have modified the answer to negative-accentuated strength training. And now I certainly have to include the impacts of sipping ice water throughout the day, the new discoveries related to brown fat and the cold plunge, plus the thermodynamics formula of transferring fat, killing it, and finally keeping it off.

But today, as I reexamine all my successful programs, I see clearly that the real power, the authentic synergy, is in the mix:

- Reduced-calorie, carbohydrate-rich eating plan
- Negative-accentuated strength training

- Superhydration
- Heat and cold transfer

Remember: 1 + 1 + 1 + 1 = 16. That's the synergy of combining a correct eating plan, proper negative-accentuated training, superhydration, and heat and cold transfer into a successful blend.

On page 22, this winning team is shown graphically in six circles under the heading "Thermodynamic Synergy." You'll notice that the big circle encloses four times the area of the smaller circles. That's thermodynamic synergy. You can now visualize why Killing Fat is such a powerful program for body transformation. You not only lose fat, but you build muscle simultaneously . . . all at an accelerating rate.

With thermodynamic synergy in full bloom, that inner circle, labeled "Killing Fat," will expand to the size of the outer circle. That's a major goal. When it happens, there will be no stopping you and your transforming body.

Now imagine the *inverse* of the diagram: each of your fat cells shrinking synergistically from the size of the biggest circle down to the size of the smallest circle. On a microscopic level, that's what is happening inside the majority of your fat cells.

Here's to you getting the right combination . . . for a life filled with thermodynamic synergy.

Doggone It!

Sometimes the concept of thermodynamic fat transfer is understood better by observing a behavior that most dogs display.

Ever have your dog misbehave inside your home? If so, you might chase the mutt outside, shouting, "Out, dog, out!" But once outside, your dog whimpers and hangs around the door, waiting impatiently to get back inside.

Fat, once it leaves your body, reacts like a misbehaving dog put outside. It paces around nearby, waiting for the opportunity to get back in. Remember, you really don't lose fat—you only *transfer* the heat from it. But where do you transfer the heat to? Fat goes outside into the environment . . . and it usually wants back in.

Once in the environment, however—the warm gases, primarily carbon dioxide—can be used by living plants that transfer it back into the environment, or transform it into food, where it can be used again by animals, including you.

Such is thermodynamics and the interchange of fat, heat, calories, and energy. Thanks to Albert Einstein, it's a fusion of Biology 101 and Physics 460. Again, you don't lose fat—you relocate, displace, shuffle, and convert it into the ecosystem.

But it's always ready to transition back inside your body. *You must destroy it.*

Death to Fat

You kill fat by being aware, vigilant, and ever-mindful of thermo-dynamics. Fire up your muscles. Superhydrate your systems. Shiver more. Consume nutritionally dense foods, in moderation. Get extra rest and sleep.

Unlock your life to synergy. Now add thermodynamics to it.

If necessary, transfer your heat—repeatedly—until you get your leanness, strength, and metabolism just right. Keep your guard up and be ready to act and react. Understand the conditions. Be alert.

To keep your transformed body *permanently* lean and strong, you must have the discipline to apply the guidelines in this book, not only for six weeks or twelve weeks—but for the rest of your life. Remember, as you continue, the process does get less complex—thanks to thermo-dynamic synergy.

Look often at the before-and-after pictures and reexamine the stories of the individuals who have successfully kept their bodies lean. Each one has beaten the odds, with unusual discipline and extra muscle. Don't forget that muscle adds fire, action, and stoke to your metabolism.

Appreciate often that thermodynamics is based on unchanging scientific laws. There will never be an easy way to go from fatness to leanness.

Recognize, too, that your body demands before it rewards. You have to *do* before you can *have*. When you're *tough* on yourself, life becomes more purposeful, more productive, and, ultimately, less taxing. That's the essence of synergy.

The rules I've challenged you with in this book are seldom glamorous and sometimes hard to face. But practicing those guidelines eventually leads to the lifestyle changes that must occur for year-after-year permanence.

Remain Unyielding

Stay the course. Hurl defiance. Stand your ground. With preparation and persistence, you can *do* and you can *have*.

Excess fat: Be gone! Stay gone!

Your quest for thermodynamic synergy is being fulfilled. You've earned the rewards.

Blast. Destroy. *Kill.*
Conquer. Enjoy. *Share.*

BIBLIOGRAPHY

Alviar, Carlos L., and others. "Marriage Linked to Lower Heart Disease Risks in Study of More Than 3.5 Million Adults." Science Daily, March 28, 2014.

Bavishi, Avni, and others. "A Chapter a Day: Association of Book Reading with Longevity." *Social Science and Medicine* 164 (Sept. 2016): 44–48.

Boschmann, Michael, and others. "Water-Induced Thermogenesis." *Journal of Clinical Endocrinology & Metabolism* 88, no. 12 (2003): 6015–19.

Carlson, Tyler. "Top 10 Fattest Countries in the World—2017 List." Gazette Review, April 15, 2017.

Chetty, Raj, and others. "The Association Between Income and Life Expectancy in the United States, 2001–2014." *Journal of the American Medical Association* 315, no. 16 (Apr. 2016): 1750–66.

Consumer Reports. "6 Truths About a Gluten-Free Diet." January 2015.

Darden, Ellington. *The Nautilus Diet.* Boston: Little, Brown, 1987.

———. *Living Longer Stronger.* New York: Perigee/Berkley, 1995.

———. *A Flat Stomach ASAP.* New York: Simon & Schuster/Pocket, 1998.

———. *The Body Fat Breakthrough.* New York: Rodale, 2014.

———. *Tighten Your Tummy in 2 Weeks.* New York: Rodale, 2015.

Davis, Lisa M., and others. "Efficacy of a Meal Replacement Diet Plan Compared to a Food-Based Diet Plan after a Period of Weight Loss and Weight Maintenance." *Nutrition Journal* 9 (Mar. 2010): 11.

Doheny, Kathleen. "The Truth About Fat," WebMD, July 13, 2009.

Elliot, Danielle. "The Doctor Who Coaches Athletes on Sleep," *The Atlantic*, April 23, 2014.

Fildes, Alison, and others. "Probability of an Obese Person Attaining Normal Body Weight: Cohort Study Using Electronic Health Records." *American Journal of Public Health* 105, no. 9 (2015): 54–9.

Frestedt, Joy L., and others. "Meal Replacement Beverages Twice a Day in Overweight and Obese Adults." *Current Nutrition and Food Science* 8, no. 4 (2012): 320–9.

Fritsch, Jane. "95% Regain Lost Weight. Or Do They?" *New York Times*, May 25, 1999.

Gibbons, Ann. "The Evolution of Diet." *National Geographic* 226, no. 3 (Sept. 2014): 34–65.

Gudzune, Kimberly A., and others. "Efficacy of Commercial Weight-Loss Programs: An Updated Systematic Review." *Annals of Internal Medicine* 162, no. 7 (2015): 501–12.

Guth, Eve. "Counting Calories as an Approach to Achieve Weight Control." *Journal of the American Medical Association* 319, no. 3 (2018): 225–6.

Guyenet, Stephen J. *The Hungry Brain*. New York: Flatiron Books, 2017.

Heller, H. Craig, and Dennis A. Grahn. "Enhanced Thermal Exchange in Humans and Practical Applications." *Disruptive Science and Technology* 1, no. 1 (2012): 1–10.

Heymsfield, Steven B., and others. "Evolving Concepts on Adjusting Human Resting Energy Expenditure Measurements for Body Size," *Obesity Reviews* 13, no. 11 (2012): 1001–14.

Jiménez-Aranda, Aroa, and others. "Melatonin Induces Browning of Inguinal White Adipose Tissue in Zucker Diabetic Fatty Rats." *Journal of Pineal Research* 55, no. 4 (Nov. 2013): 416–23.

Hall, K. D., and others. "Calorie for Calorie, Dietary Fat Restriction Results in More Body Fat Loss Than Carbohydrate Restriction in People with Obesity." *Cell Metabolism* 22, no. 3 (Sep. 2015): 427–36.

Johns Hopkins University. *The Johns Hopkins Family Health Book*. New York: HarperCollins, 1998.

Jones, Arthur. "Accentuate the Negative." *Iron Man* 32 (Jan. 1973): 30, 31, 56–59.

Keogh, Jennifer B., and Peter M. Clifton. "Meal Replacements for Weight Loss in Type 2 Diabetes in a Community Setting." *Journal of Nutrition and Metabolism* 2012 (2012). https://doi.org/10.1155/2012/918571.

Kivimaki, Mika, and others. "Body Mass Index and Risk of Dementia: Analysis of Individual-Level Data from 1.3 Million Individuals." *Alzheimer's & Dementia*, Published online: November 20, 2017.

Luoma, T. C. "The Five Different Types of Body Fat." T Nation, October 24, 2017.

———. "Tip: Sugar Is Not Addictive." T Nation, December 2, 2017.

Mah, Cheri D., and others. "The Effects of Sleep Extension on the Athletic Performance of Collegiate Basketball Players," *SLEEP* 34, no. 7 (Jul. 2011): 943–50.

Makary, Martin, and Michael Daniel. "Medical Error—The Third Leading Cause of Death in US." *British Medical Journal* 353 (2016): i2139. https://doi.org/10.1136/bmj.i2139.

Meerman, Ruben, and Andrew Brown. "When Somebody Loses Weight, Where Does the Fat Go?" *British Medical Journal* 349 (Dec. 2014): g7257. https://doi.org/10.1136/bmj.g7257.

Miller, Michael, and others. "Laughter Helps Blood Vessels Function Better." Paper presented at the Scientific Session of the American College of Cardiology, Orlando, Florida, March 7, 2005.

Moyer, Melinda Wenner. "Supercharging Brown Fat to Battle Obesity." *Scientific American*, July 15, 2014.

Mubanga, Mwenya, and others. "Dog Ownership and the Risk of Cardiovascular Disease and Death—A Nationwide Cohort Study." *Scientific Reports* 7, no. 1 (2017): 15821.

Nedeitcheva, Arlet V., and others. "Insufficient Sleep Undermines Dietary Efforts to Reduce Adiposity." *Annals of Internal Medicine* 153, no. 7 (Oct. 2010): 435–41.

GBD 2015 Obesity Collaborators. "Health Effects of Overweight and Obesity in 195 Countries over 25 Years." *New England Journal of Medicine* 377 (Jul. 2017): 13–27.

Oxenham, Simon. "Everything Is Made of Chemicals." Big Think, 2016.

Patel, Alpa V., and others. "Walking in Relation to Mortality in a Large Prospective Cohort of Older U.S. Adults." *American Journal of Preventive Medicine* 54, no. 1 (Jan. 2018): 10–19.

Pollock, M. L., and others. "Measurement of Cardio-Respiratory Fitness and Body Composition in the Clinical Setting." *Comprehensive Therapy* 6, no. 9 (Sep. 1980): 12–27.

Robinson, Matthew M., and others. "Enhanced Protein Translation Underlies Improved Metabolic and Physical Adaptations to Different Training Modes in Young and Old Humans." *Cell Metabolism* 25, no. 3 (Mar. 2017): 581–92.

Rodak, Mike. "Feeding an NFL Team for a Week," ESPN.com, October 12, 2017.

Roig, M., and others. "The Effects of Eccentric Versus Concentric Resistance Training on Muscle Strength and Mass in Healthy Adults: A Systematic Review with Meta-Analysis." *British Journal of Sports Medicine* 43 (2009): 556–68.

Shaw, M. E., and others. "Body Mass Index Is Associated with Cortical Thinning with Different Patterns in Mid- and Late-Life." *International Journal of Obesity* 42, no. 3 (Oct. 2017): 455–61.

Sifferlin, Alexandra. "The Weight Loss Trap: Why Your Diet Isn't Working." *Time*, June 5, 2017.

Sizer, Francis, and Ellie Whitney. *Nutrition Concepts & Controversies.* 14th ed. Boston: Cengage Learning, 2017.

Specter, Dina. "What It Would Look Like If Your Banana Came with an Ingredient List." *Business Insider*, June 3, 2017.

Tara, Sylvia. *The Secret Life of Fat.* New York: W. W. Norton, 2017.

Vanga, Sai Kranthi, and Vijaya Raghavan. "How Well Do Plant Based Alternatives Fare Nutritionally Compared to Cow's Milk?" *Journal of Food Science and Technology* 55, no. 1 (Jan. 2018): 10–20.

Winett, Richard A., and Ralph N. Carpinelli. "Potential Health-Related Benefits of Resistance Training." *Preventive Medicine* 33, no. 5 (No. 2001): 503–13.

Xu, Booji, and Xiangyang Xie. "Neurotrophic Factor Control of Satiety and Body Weight." *Nature* 17, no. 5 (May 2016): 282–92.

Wang, S., and others. "Resveratrol Induces Brown-Like Adipocyte Formation in White Fat Through Activation of AMP-Activated Protein Kinase." *International Journal of Obesity* 39, no. 6 (Jun. 2015): 967–76.

Whitten, Ari, and Wade Smith. *The Low Carb Myth.* Lexington, KY: Archangel Ink, 2015.

ACKNOWLEDGMENTS

I want to recognize and thank the following people who helped me in the *Killing Fat* research and book project:

Joe Cirulli and his staff at Gainesville Health & Fitness. Since 1985, Joe has been open to any research idea I wanted to test and compare—and I've done dozens of them with members at his Main Club and Women's Club.

Jeanenne Darden, my lean, strong, beautiful wife, for helping me throughout this project. Our children—**Amy, Sarah, Tyler,** and **Larah**—for their amazing teamwork.

Jeff Csatari, executive editor of the 2015 *Men's Health* book group at Rodale, who paved the way for *Killing Fat* to be published.

Erin Niumata, my literary agent, for her patience in staying on top of each step, twist, problem, and achievement.

Paul Privette of Footstone Photography in Gainesville, Florida, for taking the informative photos for Chapter 9.

Michael Ajazi of Clearwater, Florida, for being in tip-top shape for the exercise photos in Chapter 9.

Billie DeNunzio of Gainesville, Florida, for her chef and recipe skills applied in Chapter 12.

Michael Spillane of Gainesville, Florida, for his enthusiastic work ethic.

Tom Hall of Colorado Springs, Colorado, and T-Nation.com for his consistency in preparing the before-and-after digital photography.

At Rodale Books: **Alyse Diamond,** the associate editorial director, who supervised the *Killing Fat* manuscript with crisp editing and precision; associate editor **Michele Eniclerico** for her second half command and steady focus; **Elizabeth Rendfleisch** for her art direction and stunning design; and **Ivy McFadden** for her copyediting and attention to details.

My sincere appreciation to the more than 1,800 people who I've personally trained over the last fifty years...and especially the thirty-seven individuals who I featured in the comparison photographs throughout *Killing Fat*.

INDEX

A

Academy of Nutrition and Dietetics, 69
addiction, to sugar, 62–63
aerobic activity, 73
alcohol, 50, 69, 211, 221
ambient temperature, 43–44, 225–226, 228–229
American Council on Exercise, 254
American Heart Association, 59, 69
American Institute for Cancer Research, 59
American Society of Addiction Medicine, 63
Arnold, Jeff, 248
Asmussen, Erling, 76

B

backloading, 31–40
    about, 31–32
    fat loss and, 36–38
    muscular growth and, 33–35
    relaxed vs. contracted test, 38–40
    30–10–30 technique, 32–33

beef
    Skirt Steak Salad, 171
    Sweet & Sour Thai Beef Salad, 160–161
belly bloat, 47–50
belly fat, 43
beverages. *See also* hydration; Super Smoothies
    alcohol, 50, 69, 211, 221
    carbonated beverages, 49–50
    water, 217–223
Blake, Ted, 312
blood sugar metabolism, 211, 226–227, 228
body fat
    about, 25–26, 44–46
    brown fat metabolism, 43–44, 224–229
    calories-per-day guidelines for, 70–71, 140
    fat cell characteristics, 46–47
    fat loss vs. weight loss, 19, 36–40
    hanging skin and, 235, 237
    ideal percentage, 137, 254

body fat (*cont.*)
  love handles, 209–210, 259–260
  measurements, 134–137, 253–254
  thermodynamics and, 13–18, 44, 50
  types of, 41–44, 209–210, 224–229
The Body Fat Breakthrough (Darden), 78–79
body measurements, 134–137, 253–254
bottled water, 221–222
brain health, 54–55
Brown, Andrew, 16–17
Brown, Edwin "Truck," 290–291
Brownell, Kelly, 28
brown fat metabolism, 43–44, 224–229
butt fat, 42–43, 209–210

C

caffeine, 221
calories
  defined, 15–16
  fat loss vs. weight loss, 19, 36–37
  guidelines for, 19, 65, 70–71, 140, 189–190
  low-calorie dieting, 19, 30
  sleeping while burning calories, 241–242
carbohydrates
  about, 65, 250–251
  brown fat metabolism and, 227–228
  calories per gram, 15
  guidelines for, 69, 73, 251
  as hydrated carbons, 68–69, 252
  importance of, 67, 72–73, 270–271
low-carbohydrate dieting, 18–19, 72–73, 250–251, 252
  vs. proteins, 19, 66–69, 250–251
  sources of, 68
carbonated beverages, 49–50
cardio-aerobic activity, 73
Carnes, Nannette, 260
cereals, 173–175, 179
chewing gum, 48–49
circadian rhythm, 244–245
Circles of Synergy, 21–22, 293. *See also* thermodynamic synergy
Cirulli, Joe, 4, 78, 181, 183, 186–187
cold-plunge protocol
  about, 230–232
  alternatives, 236, 256–257
  hanging skin and, 237
  research and results, 44
  tips, 233–234, 235–236, 257
concentric muscle action, 75–76, 195
conduction, 232, 257
convection, 232–233
Cook-at-Home Eating Option, 153–180
  about, 139–140, 153–154; bonus meals, 179–180
  Apple Pie Oatmeal, 175
  Black Bean Veggie Patties, 155
  Blueberry Banana Oatmeal, 174
  Chickpea Salad with Couscous and Spiced Carrots, 177
  Classic Derby Cobb Salad with Turkey Cutlets, 158–159
  Deviled Egg Sandwich, 178
  Egg White Omelet, 172
  Grilled Lemon & Rosemary Shrimp, 167
  Grilled Mahimahi, 180

Homemade Granola, 173
Pear & Blue Cheese Pita, 176
Quick & Easy Meatless "Chicken" Dinner, 166
Quinoa Pilaf with Pistachios, 157
Robust Turkey Meatball Soup, 156
Rosemary Roasted Chicken & Sweet Potatoes, 170
Shirataki Shrimp Scampi Fettuccine, 164–165
Skirt Steak Salad, 171
Spaghetti Squash Turkey Bolognese, 168–169
Spinach Salad, 180
Sweet & Sour Thai Beef Salad, 160–161
Zesty Lime Shrimp Salad, 162–163
cravings, 63
Curry, Steph, 264–265
Czeisler, Charles, 243–244

D
dairy products, 48, 61, 69
Davis, Lisa M., 183
Deely, Austin, ii
dehydration. *See* hydration
depot fat, 41–43
Dietary Reference Intakes (DRI), 56, 251
dog owners, 274

E
eating plan, 59–65, 66–73. *See also* Cook-at-Home Eating Option; No-Fuss Eating Option
about, 17, 59, 69
for belly bloat, 47–48, 50
breakfast, importance of, 249

brown fat metabolism and, 227–228
calorie guidelines, 19, 65, 70–71, 140, 189–190
carbohydrates and, 65, 66–69, 72–73. *See also* carbohydrates
discipline and, 71–73, 209, 210, 249
false hunger and, 249–250
fiber-rich diet, 210–211
food groupings, 60–61
genetics and, 37, 209–210
junk foods, 63
lifestyle guidelines, 211–212, 267–274, 285–286
meal frequency, 71, 271
meal plans, 189–193, 213
meal size and portion control, 24, 70–71, 144, 153, 271
nutrients, defined, 60
processed foods, 64–65, 143–144
sugar guidelines, 61–63, 67, 68–69
tips, 140, 272, 273
eccentric muscle action, 75–76, 195
eggs
Classic Derby Cobb Salad with Turkey Cutlets, 158–159
Deviled Egg Sandwich, 178
Egg White Omelet, 172
Scrambled Eggs, 179
Einstein, Albert, 12–13
elderly, 244, 260–262
essential fat, 41–42, 43
essential nutrients, 60
estrogen, 42
evaporation, 226, 232–233
exercising. *See* aerobic activity; free weights; negative-accentuated strength training; strength-training machines

F

false hunger, 249–250
fat loss. *See* Killing Fat programs
fats (dietary), 15, 19, 59, 69
fiber-rich diet, 210–211
15–15–15 muscle-building
    technique, 79–80
Fildes, Alison, 28–29
firefighters' fat loss challenge,
    203–205
fish and shellfish
    Grilled Lemon & Rosemary
        Shrimp, 167
    Grilled Mahimahi, 180
    Shirataki Shrimp Scampi
        Fettuccine, 164–165
    Zesty Lime Shrimp Salad, 162–163
Fisher, James, 20–21
Flanagan, Jim, 82
A Flat Stomach ASAP (Darden), 207
food and nutrition. *See* eating plan
food scale recommendations, 140
Freedman, Larry, 10, 20
free weights, 84–108
    about, 83; brown fat metabolism
        and, 226; before exercising,
        257–258; muscle-building-only
        programs, 56, 238–240, 252–253,
        262; post-exercise, 235–236, 258;
        routines, 199–202, 213
    barbell bench press, 90–92
    barbell curl, 93–94
    barbell overhead press, 97–99
    barbell squat, 84–86
    dumbbell hammer curl, 95–96
    dumbbell squat, 87–89
    dumbbell triceps extension,
        100–101
    negative-only chin-up, 107–108
    negative-only dip, 105–106
    sit-up on declined board,
        102–104, 258–259
Frestedt, Joy L., 183
Fritsch, Jane, 27–28
frozen, microwavable meals, 142,
    143–144, 146, 153
fructose, 62
fruits
    about, apples, 227–228
    Apple Pie Oatmeal, 175
    Blueberry Banana Oatmeal,
        174
    Pear & Blue Cheese Pita, 176
    smoothies with, 184–186
full-body photographs, guidelines,
    138–139

G

Gaffney, Barrie, 26
gas, in digestive tract, 47–50
Gavarrete, Elijah, 37–39
genetics, of fat loss, 37, 46, 209–210
Gentry, Joe, 132
glucose, 45, 211, 226–227, 229,
    250–251
Gonzalez, Guillermo, 184, 187
Greenberg, Will, 272–273
growth hormone (GH), 5, 196–197
gum chewing, 48–49

H

hanging skin, 235, 237
Hastay, Ian, 52–54
Hastay, Noah, 52
Hastay, Travis, 52–54
Hedges, Sarah, 310
Hill, Marlene, 229
honey, 62

hormones
    fat cell production of, 42, 45
    meal size and production of, 71
    sleep cycle and, 226, 241, 243, 245
    strength training and, 5, 17,
        196–197, 243
hospitalizations, 274
Howell, Ken, 8
hunger, 24, 42, 45, 219, 241, 245,
    249–250
hydrated carbons, 68–69, 252
hydration
    about, 25, 73
    belly bloat reduction through, 48
    guidelines for, 69, 255–256
    hanging skin and, 237
    ice-cold water, 217–223, 255–256
    superhydration, 17, 211, 218–222,
        237, 271

I

inertia, law of, 194–195
inherited fat, 41–42
insoluble fiber, 210–211
insulin, 71, 197
insulin-like growth factor 1 (IGF-1),
    196–197
interleukin-6 (IL-6), 196–197
interleukin-15 (IL-15), 196–197

J

Jones, Arthur, 1–3, 76, 242
junk foods, 63

K

ketone bodies, 251
Killing Fat programs. *See also*
    body fat; Cook-at-Home
    Eating Option; eating plan;

maintenance; negative-
accentuated strength training;
No-Fuss Eating Option
    about, 3–5, 17–18, 24–25
    calorie guidelines, 19, 65, 70–71,
        140, 189–190
    vs. conventional dieting programs,
        23–24, 27–30, 72–73, 252
    expectations and results, 6–7,
        29–30, 73, 263, 287–291
    formula for, 16–19, 51–55.
        See also thermodynamics;
        thermodynamic synergy
    journaling on, 275–286
    lifestyle guidelines, 211–212,
        267–274, 285–286
    muscle-building-only programs,
        56, 238–240, 252–253, 262
    physician consultations for, 133,
        262
    support during, 133–134, 273
kilocalorie, defined, 15–16
Kivimaki, Mika, 55
Knuth, Jane, 74
Kribs, William R. "Bill," 260–262

L

lactose intolerance, 48
laughter, 274
law of inertia, 194–195
Lean Cuisine frozen meals, 142,
    143–144, 146
lemons and limes, with water, 221
lifestyle guidelines, 211–212,
    267–274, 285–286
love handles, 209–210, 259–260
low-calorie dieting, 19, 30
low-carbohydrate dieting, 18–19,
    72–73, 250–251, 252

M

machines, strength-training. *See* negative-accentuated strength training; strength-training machines
Mah, Cheri, 243
maintenance, 264–275
  control and, 266–270
  lifestyle guidelines, 211–212, 267–274, 285–286
  overlearning, 210, 264–265, 271
  patience and, 264, 272
  practice and, 71–73, 270
  tips, 268–272
marriage, 274
Mayo Clinic Libraries, 64
McGinley, Julie, 138
meal planning. *See* Cook-at-Home Eating Option; eating plan; No-Fuss Eating Option
measurements (body), 134–137, 253–254
mechano growth factor (MGF), 196–197
Medary, Branden, 35, 141
Medary, Chris, 34–36
Medary, Max, 35
Meerman, Ruben, 16–17
Meisner, Ashley, 130
melatonin, 226, 245
metabolic set point, 227
microwavable, frozen meals, 142, 143–144, 146, 153
multivitamins, 140
muscle-building-only programs, 56, 238–240, 252–253, 262
muscle mass. *See also* negative-accentuated strength training
  brain health and, 54–55
  hanging skin and, 235, 237
  muscle gain determination, 134–137, 196–197
  protein vs. carbohydrates for, 66

N

National Institutes of Health, 251
The Nautilus Diet (Darden), 206, 207
Nedeltcheva, Arlet, 241
negative-accentuated strength training. *See also* backloading; free weights; strength-training machines
  about, 5, 17, 24–25, 75–77, 194–196
  brown fat metabolism during, 226
  exercises and routines. *See* free weights; strength-training machines
  15–15–15 technique, 79–80
  hormone production and, 196–197
  muscle-building-only programs, 56, 238–240, 252–253, 262
  research on, 76–77
  30–10–30 technique, 32–33, 80–81, 83, 194–195
  30–30–30 technique, 79
  tips, 73, 197–199, 235–236, 257–258, 271
  X-Force equipment, 77–79
negative muscle action, 76, 194–195
Newton's law of inertia, 194–195
No-Fuss Eating Option, 142–152
  about, 142–143; bonus meals, 179–180; frozen, microwavable meals, 142, 143–144, 146,

153; menus for weeks 1
and 2, 147–149; menus for
weeks 3 through 6, 150–152;
recommendations, 139–140;
results with, 144; shopping list,
145–146
cereals, 179
Grilled Mahimahi, 180
Scrambled Eggs, 179
Spinach Salad, 180
nutrition. *See* eating plan

O

O'Connell, Tom, 203–205
older adults, 244, 260–262
overlearning, 210, 264–265, 271

P

Pare, Wayne, 246
patience, 264, 272
peanut butter
–Berry Blitz smoothie, 185
and jelly sandwiches, 272
photographs, guidelines for,
138–139
pinch test, 135–136, 137
Poole, Shane, 238–240, 253
portion control, 24, 70–71, 144, 153,
271
positive muscle action, 76, 194–195
poultry
Classic Derby Cobb Salad with
Turkey Cutlets, 158–159
Robust Turkey Meatball Soup,
156
Rosemary Roasted Chicken &
Sweet Potatoes, 170
Spaghetti Squash Turkey
Bolognese, 168–169

Powell, Clifton, 235, 237
processed foods, 64–65, 143–144,
146, 153
proteins
calories per gram, 15
vs. carbohydrates, 19, 66–69,
250–251
guidelines for, 69, 70

R

radiation, 233, 257
Rapport, Jordan, 33–34
recipes. *See* Cook-at-Home Eating
Option; No-Fuss Eating
Option; Super Smoothies;
specific recipe types
refined-flour products, 68–69
Rivera, Edgardo, 214
Roberts, Storm, 265–270
Rodriguez, Angel, iii, 259–260,
289–290
Roig, Marc, 76–77
room temperature, 43–44, 225–226,
228–229

S

Sagan, Carl, 18–19, 65
salads
Chickpea Salad with Couscous
and Spiced Carrots, 177
Classic Derby Cobb Salad with
Turkey Cutlets, 158–159
Skirt Steak Salad, 171
Spinach Salad, 180
Sweet & Sour Thai Beef Salad,
160–161
Zesty Lime Shrimp Salad,
162–163
salt intake, 47, 48

Schendel, Harold E., 66, 67–69
Shaw, Jeff, 275–286
Shaw, Marnie, 54–55
sibling fat-loss challenge, 52–54,
    207–209, 212
skipping meals, 249
sleeping and resting, 238–245
    about, 73, 211, 238–240
    belly bloat reduction and, 50
    guidelines, 228–229, 240–241,
        244
    hormones and, 226, 241, 243,
        245
    naps, 243–244
    research and results, 241–242,
        244–245
Smith, Bob, 12, 311
Smith, Gary, 58
smoothies. *See* Super Smoothies
soluble fiber, 210–211
Spalding, Ken, 71–73
Spencer, Candace, 216
Spratt, Allison, 207–209, 212
Spratt, Doug, 206, 209–212,
    259–260
Stansfield, Jennifer, 49
Stare, Fredrick, 61
strength-training machines
    about: brown fat metabolism
        during, 226; before exercising,
        257–258; post-exercise,
        235–236, 258; routines,
        200–202, 213
    abdominal crunch, 127–129,
        258–259
    calf raise, 118–120
    chest press, 121–122
    lat machine pulldown, 123–124
    lat machine pushdown, 125–126

leg curl, 112–114
leg extension, 109–111
leg press, 115–117
Stunkard, Albert, 28
subcutaneous fat, 41–42
sugars, 61–63, 67, 68–69, 221
superhydration, 17, 211, 218–222,
    237, 271
Super Smoothies, 181–188
    about: blender choices, 182–183;
        calorie count for, 183; prepare
        and adapt, 186–187; for
        teenagers, 187–188; tips,
        181–182
    Apple a Day, 185–186
    Avocado Go Go, 186
    Bananarama, 185
    Dark Chocolate Delight, 185
    Peanut Butter–Berry Blitz, 185
    Purple Heaven, 186
    Strawberry-Pistachio Punch,
        184
synergy. *See* thermodynamic
    synergy

T
tap water, 221–222
teenagers
    gradual muscle growth for,
        34–35
    sleep requirements, 244
    smoothies for, 187–188
teeth, brushing and flossing, 211
television, 211
temperature, ambient, 43–44,
    225–226, 228–229
thermodynamics, 11–22. *See also*
    thermodynamic synergy
    about, 12–13, 25–26

calorie, defined, 15–16
defined, 5
of fat transfer, 13–18, 44, 50
Killing Fat formula and, 16–19,
    51–55
muscles and, 27
transfer, defined, 14–15
thermodynamic synergy. *See also*
    cold-plunge protocol; sleeping
    and resting
about, 21–22, 51–52, 292–295
for belly bloat, 50
for body fat transference, 13–18,
    44, 50
brain health and, 54–55
brown fat metabolism, 43–44,
    224–229
Circles of Synergy, 21–22, 293
defined, 51
Killing Fat formula and, 16–19,
    51–55
water, ice-cold, 217–223. *See also*
    hydration
thermostat, setting, 228–229
thigh fat, 42–43, 209–210
30–10–30 muscle-building
    technique. *See* free weights;
    negative-accentuated strength
    training; strength-training
    machines
30–30–30 muscle building
    technique, 79
Thulin, Mats, 77–78
Truttmann, Darin, i
Tucker, Ted, 217–218, 222
turkey. *See* poultry
20–10–20 muscle-building
    technique, 83

U
U.S. Department of Agriculture
    (USDA), 60–61, 62

V
vegetarian dishes
    Black Bean Veggie Patties, 155
    Quick & Easy Meatless "Chicken"
        Dinner, 166
    Quinoa Pilaf with Pistachios, 157
Viator, Casey, 39–40
visceral fat, 43

W
Walker, Joe, 56, 252–253
warm-up routine, 257–258
water, 217–223. *See also* hydration
weight loss, fat loss vs., 19, 36–40
white fat, 42–43, 224, 227
women
    belly bloat and, 47
    body fat percentage, ideal, 137,
        254
    butt and thigh fat, 42–43,
        209–210
    calories-per-day guidelines, 70
    exercising techniques for, 79–80
    expectations, 5, 6, 37
    genetics and, 37, 46, 209–210
    results, 26, 49, 74, 130, 138, 216,
        229
Woody, Javier, 230–231
work ethic, 71–73, 266–270
Wright, Will, 187–188
Wykle, Tom, 288

X
X-Force equipment, 77–79

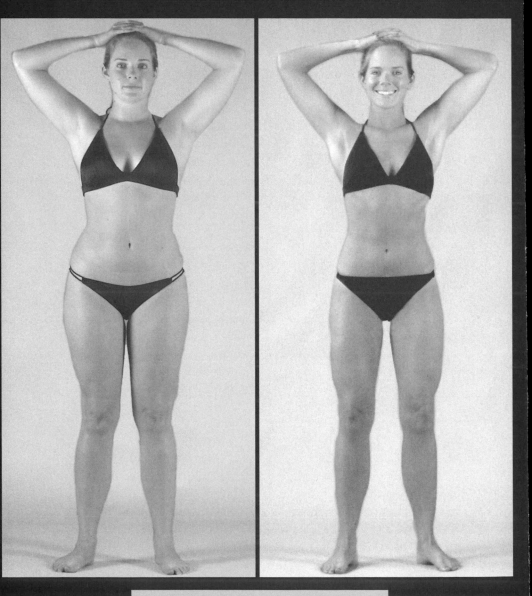

158.6 pounds   **135.1** pounds

SARAH HEDGES, age 25, height 5'7.5"
AFTER 12 WEEKS
26.86 pounds of fat loss
6 inches off waist, **6.125** inches off thighs
3.36 pounds of muscle gain

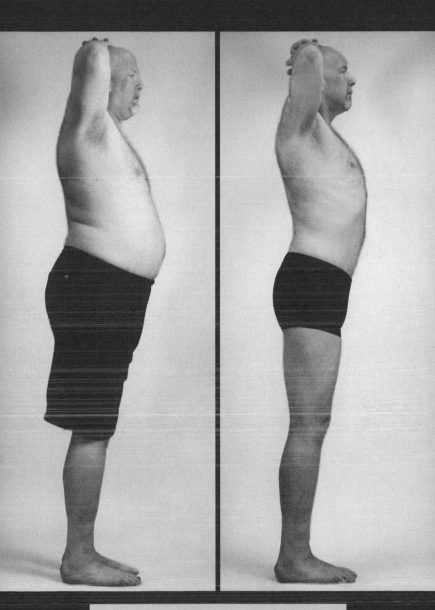

302 pounds   241 pounds

BOB SMITH, age 51, height 6'7"
AFTER 80 DAYS
80 pounds of fat loss
11 inches off waist
19 pounds of muscle gain

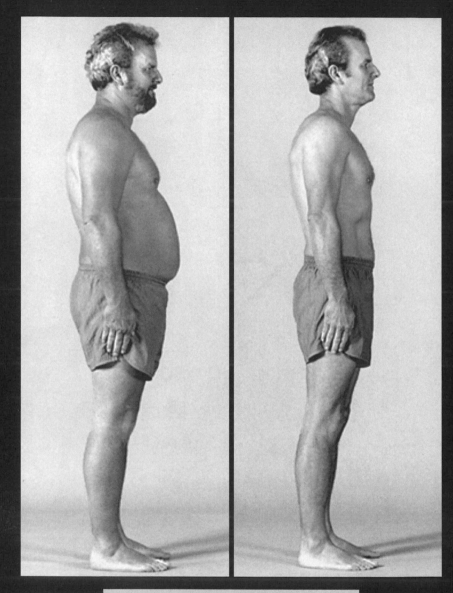

221.5 pounds   **157.25** pounds

TED BLAKE, age 41, height 5'7.25"
AFTER 20 WEEKS
67.75 pounds of fat loss
10.25 inches off waist
3.5 pounds of muscle gain